The Yoga of Niguma

THE YOGA OF NIGUMA

TIBETAN PRACTICES FOR
A LUMINOUS MIND

His Eminence Kalu Rinpoche
with Michele Loew

Illustrated by Mia Scarpetta

Foreword by His Holiness the Dalai Lama

Wisdom Publications
132 Perry Street
New York, NY 10014 USA
wisdom.org

© 2025 Kalu Rinpoche and Michele Loew
All rights reserved.

No part of this book may be reproduced in any form or by any means, electronic or mechanical, including photography, recording, or by any information storage and retrieval system or technologies now known or later developed, without permission in writing from the publisher.

Library of Congress Cataloging-in-Publication Data is available.
LCCN 2024060708 (print) | LCCN 2024060709 (ebook)

ISBN 978-1-61429-952-3   ebook ISBN 978-1-61429-976-9

29 28 27 26 25
5 4 3 2 1

Illustrations by Mia Scarpetta. Cover and interior design by Gopa & Ted2, Inc.

Printed on acid-free paper that meets the guidelines for permanence and durability of the Production Guidelines for Book Longevity of the Council on Library Resources.

Printed in Canada.

The information provided in this book is for educational purposes only and is not intended to replace professional medical advice. You should consult with a healthcare provider before implementing any new practices or changes to your health and exercise regimen, including the practices discussed in this book. The authors and publisher are providing this book and its contents on an "as is" basis and make no representations or warranties of any kind with respect to this book or its contents. The authors and publisher disclaim any and all such representations and warranties, including but not limited to warranties of merchantability or fitness for a particular purpose.

Contents

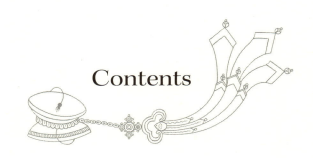

List of Practices	ix
Foreword by His Holiness the Dalai Lama	xiii
Preface	xv

PART 1: Introducing Niguma Yoga

1. The Lineage of the Practices	3

PART 2: Preparation of Mind and Body and Practical Guidance for the Yogic Lifestyle

2. Preparation of the Mind	9
3. Yogic Lifestyle: Health, Safety, and Practical Guidance	21

PART 3: The Yoga of Niguma

4. Building Your Niguma Yoga Practice	31
5. The Yoga of Niguma Sequences: Illustrations and Instructions	49
6. Conclusion	147
Acknowledgments	151
Appendix: Supportive Hatha Yoga Postures	157
Additional Resources	167
About the Authors	169

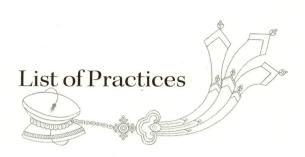

List of Practices

Foundational Vajra Posture and Breathing	32
Vajra Fists	33
Arrow Breath in Preparation for Vase Breath Before a Pose	33
Vase Breathing	34
Arrow Breath upon Completion of a Pose	37
Yogic Breathing	38
Constructive Rest Pose	39
Seated Yoga Breathing for Diaphragmatic Awareness	42
Viloma Pranayama	43
Pranayama Utilizing 1:2 Ratio	44
Niguma Yoga Sequence 1: Freeing the Knots in the Channels	49
Seated Twist 1	51
Seated Twist 2: Ardha Matsyendrasana (Half Lord of the Fishes)	52
Niguma Yoga Sequence 2: Straightening the Channels	55
Shik (Breaking the Posture)	55
Bep (Controlled Fall or Mindful Transition to a Seat)	55
Virabhadrasana 2 (Warrior 2)	60
Niguma Yoga Sequence 3: Gathering into the Uma	63
Niguma Yoga Sequence 4: Spreading Out Through the Channels	65
Janu Sirsasana (Head-to-Knee Pose)	68

Niguma Yoga Sequence 5: Standing and Spreading Through the Channels	71
Niguma Yoga Sequence 6: Moving the Limbs	73
Niguma Yoga Sequence 7: Pressing Down from the Upper Body	75
Niguma Yoga Sequence 8: One Leg	77
Niguma Yoga Sequence 9: Two Legs	79
Niguma Yoga Sequence 10: Twisting	81
Seated Crescent Pose	84
Standing Crescent Moon Pose	85
Niguma Yoga Sequence 11: Like a Small Child	87
Niguma Yoga Sequence 12: Falling	89
Figure Four Pose	92
Figure Four Pose at a Wall	92
Baddha Konasana (Bound Angle Pose)	93
Niguma Yoga Sequences 13 and 14: Opening the Uma	97
Opposite Arm-Leg Extension	100
Shalabhasana (Locust Pose)	101
Niguma Yoga Sequence 15: Entering the Uma	103
Niguma Yoga Sequence 16: Drawing Up the Uma	107
Niguma Yoga Sequence 17: Gathering into the Uma 2	109
Niguma Yoga Sequence 18 : Yoga Practice that Dispels the Kleshas (Addictions)	111
Niguma Yoga Sequence 19: Dispelling Agitation	115
Niguma Yoga Sequence 20: Overpowering the Harmful	119
Niguma Yoga Sequence 21: Dispelling Aggression and Aversion with the Mudra of Akshobhya and Dispelling Pride with the Mudra of Amitabha	123
Niguma Yoga Sequence 22: Dispelling Desire	127
Ardha Navasana (Half-Boat Pose and Hollow Body)	130

Niguma Yoga Sequence 23: The Lesser Descent of Supreme Bliss	131
Garudasana (Eagle Pose)	133
Lying Down Shoulder Stretch	135
Niguma Yoga Sequence 24: The Greater Descent of Supreme Bliss that Dispels Greed	137
Niguma Yoga Sequence 25: Shaking "Ha!"	143
Vajra Posture (Lotus Pose)	157
Variations of the Figure Four Pose	159
Seated Figure Four Pose	159
Supta Padangusthasana (Reclined Leg Stretching on the Back)	160
Janu Sirsasana (Head-to-Knee Pose)	162
Supta Eka Pada Raja Kapotasana (Reclined Pigeon Pose)	164

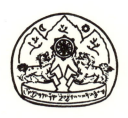

THE DALAI LAMA

Foreword

THE TEACHINGS OF NIGUMA, an Indian yogini, inspired the founding of the Shangpa Kagyu lineage of Tibetan Buddhism, of which Kalu Rinpoche is a lineage holder. The previous Kalu Rinpoche, who passed away in 1989, was a learned and respected master.

Continuing his predecessor's legacy, the current Kalu Rinpoche has now written a book, *The Yoga of Niguma*, explaining the practice with clear instructions. It is a practice that involves the body, breath, and mind, and as related in the book, it is a powerful means for achieving physical and mental well-being.

Rinpoche makes clear that the yoga of Niguma is motivated by lovingkindness, with the aim of achieving peace of mind and sharing the happiness that entails.

May all who seek to apply themselves sincerely be blessed with success, for the benefit of others and themselves.

25 November 2024

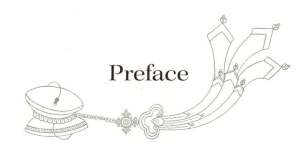

Preface

THE YOGA OF NIGUMA can bring you to the highest level of joy, bliss, and contentment. Even though this practice developed within Buddhism over hundreds of years, you don't need to consider yourself a Buddhist to engage in it and experience its tremendous benefits; a humanistic outlook is all you need. Our body and mind typically perceive reality through the senses: hearing, smell, sight, touch, taste, and thought. If you take some distance and begin to divest from the senses—something that might seem counterintuitive—you will not lose your mind and descend into a delusional state. Instead, you will be ready to realize a lucid, blissful clarity. If Niguma yoga is practiced with proper guidance as written in this book, you will experience enhanced contentment and a peaceful attitude. Try doing these postures for a few hours—that may be all you need to get an initial taste of calmness and clarity, the subjective states we all seek and can gain through this practice. Tens of millions of people have taken up the practice of hatha yoga. To me, this demonstrates how much we all want to be elevated beyond our limitations, how much we all want to feel healthy and positive. This physical benefit *and* calmness and clarity is open to you in the practice of the yoga of Niguma. However, that is just the beginning. For those who are ready for dynamic change or who seek wholesale personal transformation, deeper and more subtle experiences await.

Furthermore, for those of you who engage with this practice from a Buddhist perspective, you may additionally experience a nondualistic state of mind with this yoga. Especially once mastery over the breath is gained, you eventually see that the self-existent mind is an illusion. This leads you to great awareness and the ability to make sound judgment moment to moment. The result of clean, clear awareness is the liberation from deception that leads to anger, jealousy, and ignorance. Whatever arises, you are in a position to make a skillful, conclusive decision, and you may even notice a greater degree of patience. This is not to be confused with torpor or laziness; it is a patience that embodies the intimate presence of awareness. This tends to mitigate waves of anger because you are able to find more skillful means to refine actions of your body, speech, and mind as a result of this profound awareness. This can be transformative throughout your lifetime, regardless of your religion or age.

The ancient yoga of Niguma, however, has historically been a secret tradition—and it is known to be extraordinarily transcendent. In addition to offering the many benefits one would also receive through hatha yoga, this practice cultivates the subtle channels of the inner body and refines the energetic winds that flow within them. In this way, we clear internal obstacles, restore energetic circulation, and attain health through balance. Ultimately, the practitioner restores the power of one's most concentrated essence and gradually gains masterful yet gentle control of its internal movement. The fruits of the practice offer utmost clarity in one's own mind and exquisite, auspicious discernment in one's life.

Niguma's teachings and yogic methods are revered by the oldest traditions of many Vajrayana schools throughout the Himalayan region, and they are studied and practiced by scholars and meditators alike. Niguma was an exquisitely enlightened yogini who brought us this yogic tradition a thousand years ago. Many masters at that time acknowledged that the level of her realization was comparable to that of the Buddha himself.

Niguma asked her first student to promise not to allow her secret treasures to be shared with the public until seven generations had passed, and only then with precise and proper explanation. As per her condition, the first seven generations of practitioners carried out this tradition in strict secrecy. Then, once it became accessible, many Buddhist schools absorbed this tradition in earnest. Still, the yoga of Niguma remained closely held and only taught to dedicated monks during the latter part of a three-year secluded retreat.

Eventually, the previous Kalu Rinpoche began teaching *lujong* according to the lineage of Niguma—a series of yogic practices that combine movement, breathing, and awareness, the fruit of which is physical health, emotional balance, and spiritual awakening. Based on my own intense inspiration during retreat, and as a dedicated Buddhist practitioner, I was moved to follow in the footsteps of my predecessor, the previous Kalu Rinpoche, and decided to make the yoga of Niguma more accessible to the public, in large part with the many millions of hatha yoga practitioners in mind. To practice the yoga of Niguma, one is not asked to belong to any particular religion or worship any particular teacher. It is my hope and vision that this book will offer great benefit for generations to come. You, the reader, may join this living stream by taking up the practice. I wish you a very happy journey in this Niguma yoga practice. I hope our paths may cross in-person at future Niguma yoga events, wherever they may be in the world.

A Personal Journey

Childhood

As a child, I was recognized as the reincarnation of a great Buddhist teacher and given the title of "Rinpoche" by accomplished masters from different traditions: Sakya, Kagyu, Gelug, Jonang, and others. They offered me great deference as they had long held deep respect for the name of Kalu Rinpoche, as well as the teachings of Niguma and the Shangpa tradition for which my predecessor was lineage holder. Since childhood, I understood that I was expected to uphold these traditions, but I had no idea of the importance and magnitude of this responsibility.

Even though I never became a fully ordained monk with a vow of celibacy, or sexual abstinence, I have spent much of my life living in Dharma centers, monasteries, and retreat centers. At times, this was a decision made for me by my elders. However, it has also been my own choice as a human being, one that has allowed me to strengthen my study and to empower my ability to engage in extensive retreat.

When one resides in a monastery, one abides by a life that is essentially printed out for you—one must obey set rules and live by them on a daily basis. In my youth, it was not possible for me to really see anything beyond this regimen because it was before social media opened up the world, when it was uncommon to see anything on a display screen. Especially in India, the common public use of electronics came later than in Western countries. It was in that atmosphere that I went into a retreat as a youth.

Retreat
Early challenges

I entered into a three-year retreat at the age of fourteen. The timing of retreat was at the direction of my mentor; he made the recommendation because my predecessor, the previous Kalu Rinpoche, had done the same. In the retreat, I was glad that I was not subject to monastery protocols or discipline masters telling me what rules to follow. So as a young teenager, I felt liberated from the strict monastic structure I had grown up with. Although I felt liberated, there was nothing else to do but engage in Dharma practice in my square, wooden retreat box. Still, life was not as harsh and rigid as had been during my monastic studies. The atmosphere during retreat was such because the other participants, aside from myself, were adults no longer subject to the monastic discipline of children like me. Still, in reteat, one cannot walk into town, take solace in the forest, or even buy simple Indian snacks. The first year for me passed with considerable difficulty. It took great effort to steel myself to finish my practice each day as, early on, I tended toward distraction.

We began the retreat by engaging in preliminary practices, which I found quite arduous. I struggled to complete the hundred thousand prostrations. In the Vajrayana tradition, the retreat typically begins with performing one hundred thousand of each of the preliminaries (called *ngondro*): prostrations, refuge prayers and other practices for purification, consolidation of the bond with our spiritual mentor, and cultivation of generosity. All of this must be done before one may engage with advanced practice. Here, I struggled. Once our preliminary practices were complete, we progressed to the practice of the five tantric deities, the six yogas of Niguma, and then the five golden Dharmas of Niguma.

Connection with the lineage of the masters

I experienced an abrupt change during the second year of my retreat, when one day I opened a book of Niguma's teachings. Reading it, I instantly felt very much loved and understood from a spiritual standpoint. I felt deeply moved, and I experienced Niguma's intimate presence, great wisdom, and infinite compassion so deeply. It was also clear that, notwithstanding this profound opening, it was only the beginning of the spiritual work that lay ahead of me. It is a bit like seeing the sun behind the clouds. I sensed that it would require great and consistent effort. This spark led me to read further about the other great masters in the Shangpa lineage, such as Milarepa, Sukhasiddhi, Maitripa, Rahula Gupta, Khyungpo Naljor, and Mokchokpa. When I read their biographies, even though I am terrible at geography, I vividly saw in my mind's eye the climate and landscape and could clearly visualize each of their retreat locations. A few months later, I received a book from Tibet about the monastic sites of all the Shangpa masters. The photos in the book were exactly what I had visualized. I did not experience pride about this, but rather I saw this as an affirmation that gave me a greater determination to continue on the path of Niguma.

Practice of Niguma yoga

It was not until the second year of my retreat that we began to do the physical practices of Niguma yoga. Traditionally, this yoga has only been taught in the context of a deep retreat, with the practitioner having already completed the hundred thousand repetitions of each preliminary practice. A retreat master came over to teach the retreatants how to perform the specific postures. He said he was there to demonstrate the vajra cross leg in space called *dorje topbep* and how to land it. This is more difficult to perform than a simple *bep*; the practitioner must first jump into full-lotus posture in the air before descending to the mat. At that time, he said to me in front of my eighteen brothers, mockingly,

"Since you are Kalu Rinpoche, show us how special you are and demonstrate the dorje topbep." I was fifteen at the time and by far the youngest in the retreat. The others were in their twenties, thirties, and forties. What he was asking me to do was the most advanced practice and this was the first time I had ever seen it. I was so on the spot, wishing I had a way out, but I didn't. I knew that I had to draw from a place deep inside to land this posture.

I stood up, inhaled, kept air compressed in my core, and then I said to myself, "Let it be free—no attachment." My state of mind was clear, with no sense of fear. I was successful on my first attempt. When everyone else started working on this technique, I saw that it took them considerable time to master. Having succeeded with no struggle whatsoever, I felt the strong blessing of Niguma. We were told to do at least one session per day of the full set of twenty-five postures in retreat, but inspired by that initial experience, right away I started doing the Niguma yoga postures twice per day. This was a major inflection point that launched me onto the Shangpa path. I found great aspiration to become a holder of this lineage, not knowing at that point that the last Shangpa lineage holder had been my predecessor, the previous Kalu Rinpoche. I felt so touched and inspired by the Shangpa lineage that I was determined to at least have the knowledge I needed to revive it fully.

Drawn toward the Shangpa tradition

Understand that Shangpa is considered a minor lineage, a branch of the major Kagyu lineage of Vajrayana. It is a pity when minor lineages are lost or subsumed by major lineages in such a way that their wisdom is forgotten. There was a clear sense at that point in my youth that the Shangpa lineage had faded. It was no longer remembered as a distinctive lineage but a secondary branch of quite a number of other major lineages. Similarly, Shije is a minor lineage associated with Chö, or Severance, practice, and it too has been subsumed by other major lineages. Although the practices of minor lineages are studied broadly, they are not typically taken up as principal practices but secondary practices. Secondary practices are more vulnerable to being changed, overly influenced, or overlooked.

At some point, there is no one to question when changes are made and no reliable authority to whom one may ask a sincere question to refine one's practice.

I had no understanding at this point that the Shangpa tradition was in danger of fading further when I was young and in retreat, but somehow I was drawn to it so naturally and felt an obligation to uphold the lineage. After I started doing Niguma yoga, I felt great bliss intermittently over the following weeks and months. Eventually, I started to experience bliss with each session. Each day, I would do the first session with the other monks in retreat. The second session of each day I was on my own and able to proceed at my own pace; this enabled me to carefully refine the practice according to my capacity. Eventually, I found that I couldn't take a day off, regardless of sun or rain. There was an incredible force within. It felt like the blessing of Niguma was so strong that I couldn't stop.

Fruits of clarity

I did not get sick or injured, not even with a cold, for the two years I remained in retreat. With each session of Niguma yoga I felt greater clarity and strength of mind, as well as a peaceful sense of calm abiding without grasping. Through this one practice, all other practices became clear. The effects of Niguma yoga felt pervasive and carried over to my practice of Six-Arm Mahakala, Green Tara, and long-life pujas.

Over time, I felt extraordinarily clear with strong awareness. I had the sense that I was simultaneously understanding and truly experiencing the subtle Dharma, and it brought tears to my eyes. It gave me a sense of the Dharma not just at a surface level but a profound level, helping me understand the great masters and protectors of the lineage. When I reached that stage of experience, my clothes became less important, regardless of the dirt I might see around my neck. My sense of engagement with the physical space around me had drastically reduced. My impulse to walk around and desire to feel this or that waned. This shift grew and strengthened consistently as the retreat progressed. I also found that my drive to interact with others began to fall away. Even the desires of the sense door of taste seemed to drift away.

This transformation was quite powerful. During the first year of retreat, my thoughts would wander, pondering when the retreat would end. Later, I felt that each passing day was one less day that I could remain doing this precious practice. I began wishing that each day of practice—and along with it, the experience of the bond I had with the protectors and the *dakas* and *dakinis*—the male and female representations of enlightened qualities and energies central to tantric practice—would not end. Somehow, I knew that a practitioner's life changed immensely when their retreat is over. The thought of losing even one day of practice seemed to be too much to bear. That sentiment appeared to reveal itself during that period of clear awareness, day and night.

The conclusion of the retreat

In ancient times, the yogis, as they came out of a three-year retreat, would enable others to observe their yogic abilities, and this would include secret breathing practices. The Day of Repa, as it is known in Vajrayana Buddhism, honors Milarepa, among the most revered yogis in the Kagyu lineage. He lived in the eleventh and twelfth centuries and was driven by remorse to a life of austere, ascetic practice after he harmed numerous people using black magic—an act of revenge on those who had taken his family's property and belongings. In an effort to receive teachings from the great master Marpa, he was first required to build a large stone tower, but three times after one was built, was ordered to take it down. Marpa skillfully understood that Milarepa needed to purify the karma of his previous misdeeds in this way so that the wisdom of the Dharma could take root. Milarepa is often depicted as wearing a thin cotton robe and was given the title "Repa," meaning Cotton-Clad One—he was a yogi well known for his perseverance, wisdom, and compassion.

The tradition of the Day of Repa continues to the present day. In fact, some years ago my long-time students in France completed a three-year retreat. Many of them were women in their fifth and sixth decade. On their Day of Repa, they emerged with grace, focus, and clarity on an intensely cold day with their wet sheets. Their inner transformation was unmistakable.

Seeing my own retreatants on their Day of Repa brought back clear memories of my own Day of Repa years earlier, when I was eighteen years old. I had become quite thin as I only ate a small serving of steamed cabbage each morning. That was it for the day. If I felt adventurous, I might add a few drops of soy sauce. If I felt very adventurous, I would add a small amount of oil. Without insulation, naturally, one feels the cold more readily. The other retreatants and I didn't have the opportunity to jog around to warm up. Instead, we were fully dependent on the practice itself to maintain our body heat in the elements. We wore wet sheets, dipped into ice-cold water nearby. The retreatants generated the power of the practice of inner fire by drying these sheets with their own body heat.

On my Day of the Repa, which occurred near the end of the retreat, we wore only a thin white cloth and slowly walked outside in the cold temperature, demonstrating that we had overcome the sensorial world and illusory mind. As we went outside, I knew there would be a lot people: spectators, family, friends, even future enemies. The cold air hit me at the same time as the noise of the subdued but restless crowd that had come to the monastery in India. I walked slowly outside with my eighteen Dharma brothers, chanting the names of the masters that had handed this tradition down to us. As we walked around, passing through the onlookers, there was not a moment that I lost my clean, clear awareness, the fruit of a three-year and three-month retreat. The Day of Repa was a kind of show for the spectators, replete with plenty of noise and photos. I sensed that to the observers gathered that day, I was very important, but I perceived myself as neither important nor subject to delusion. I was eighteen at that time. It was a one-day ceremony. That evening, we came back to the retreat center for our remaining six months of secluded retreat. We continued by engaging in the long-life Niguma practice and the long-life Sukhasiddhi practice until, finally, the three-year, nine-month Kalachakra retreat came to a conclusion.

Responsibilities of My Predecessor

When I came out of retreat in 2008, so many people that had met me as a child— and others that I had never met before—came to me to ask that I take over the responsibilities of the previous Kalu Rinpoche. The legacy of and responsibility for the spiritual and organizational leadership of all of the Shangpa Kagyu retreat centers started to fall to me. As I gradually worked to fulfill this role, I slowly began to lose the quality of clean, clear awareness I had gained in retreat. I was constantly traveling and involved in social engagements, and found there was little time to practice.

After twelve years back in a world full of distractions, and facing many difficulties in my role—although I facilitated improvements in the material, organizational, and administrative aspects of my centers—on a spiritual level, I found that I was holding onto the last thread of the rope.

The Pandemic and the Great Solitude

We must understand that until we reach the state of an enlightened buddha, or at least the first bodhisattva stage, we cannot take a break from our Dharma practices without a risk of backsliding in our clarity and attainments. Over the twelve years that followed my retreat, I slowly began to feel more and more drained because I had not achieved that critical threshold and had not continued practicing as intensively after the retreat. Then the COVID-19 pandemic in 2020 initiated great suffering for many throughout the world. During this difficult time, I tried to contribute as much as possible by raising funds and organizing humanitarian aid. We offered meals and medicine for sixteen thousand people in Bhutan, India, China, and Brazil.

Of course, humanitarian work is necessary and worthwhile, but working essentially as an administrator, I felt restless and knew I had to recommit myself more fully to the actual practice of Dharma. For me, the pandemic was also the beginning of a great solitude that enabled me to get back to practice. It was in 2020, during the depth of the pandemic, that I reconnected with Niguma yoga while living in Berlin. It was then that the strands of the last threads of the rope started to regenerate and multiply and braid themselves once more.

Refreshing Niguma Yoga

During the pandemic, I lived in Berlin in a small flat. Around the globe, countless beings were suffering not only from the illness that spread and harmed so many, but also from the prolonged isolation so many experienced. At one point, I sat down on the floor of my temporary residence in Berlin, looked toward the ground, and calmed my mind. Then I refreshed my skills on how to do Niguma yoga in concert with the breath. Doing so brought tears to my eyes and great memories from my retreat. I felt grateful to still be alive, in addition to being physically well and blessed with the causes and conditions to return to these precious practices. From the very first time I resumed practice in Berlin, it felt like a great void in my life had been filled again.

During that period, I had been giving teachings on meditation and the nature of the mind in a park near my home. There I befriended a couple who had been coming to the teachings: Wolfgang Stellar, a German artist, and his wife, Xiaoni-Li. As our friendship grew and my practice continued, I asked if I could use their art studio to do my yoga there. The studio was in a suburb of Berlin, and we came to an arrangement to share the space such that one of us would work in the morning until one in the afternoon. My friends kindly offered the space at no charge. It was there that I practiced the Niguma sequences three to six times per day. Within six months, I had completed the better part of one thousand sessions. Gradually, mental clarity returned, and with it the ability to see things as they truly are. Emotions stabilized, and the magnified sensations stemming from the illusion of a solidified self became tame once more. Having had such a blissful experience, I thought everyone should have an opportunity to experience this. Whether or not someone considers themself to be Buddhist, this practice would help them connect with their inner beauty and peace. Of course, it would also help those who are Buddhist practitioners excel in their spiritual understanding and realizations. It was at this time that the seed was planted, and I began considering how I might most skillfully begin to share with others what had been kept largely as a secret for so long. First, I sought appropriate permissions to teach to the public. Then, gradually, I began to offer seminars and workshops to the public. Somewhere along the way, I also had the idea for this book, which has now manifested.

Perspectives on Open Access

It is my view that Niguma yoga, combined with the proper breathing technique, counters blind faith. This practice uplifts individuals from ordinary limitations and ordinary sensorial perception. Typical limitations stem from a fixed view of self, and therefore an unrealistic perception of people and things around us. Ordinary sensorial perception is actually the greatest obstacle to subtle clarity. The practice itself clears the path to develop clarity, wisdom, and kindness.

People from all walks of life, from all cultural and religious backgrounds, are now warmly welcome to experience Niguma yoga. If approached skillfully, regardless of one's point of view or the state of one's physical body, most anyone can find a way to engage in Niguma yoga and derive benefit. I really mean it. In each seminar I teach, there are those whose physical condition dictates that they start and sometimes remain sitting in a chair at the back of the hall. That's OK.

Part of the purpose of this book is to offer insight into the nature of this discipline, its potential benefit, and how best to prepare oneself. Taking up Niguma yoga doesn't require you to convert to a new religion or step outside your existing belief system. It is also my observation that with a moderate amount of preparation, one can get started on this journey, and once underway, gain insights on any necessary adjustments that may be helpful.

GRATITUDE TO MY MENTORS

In my own case, I come from a Buddhist background. Fundamental to our tradition is sincere respect for one's teachers. However, we are not meant to follow our teachers blindly. Rather, we seek their guidance and wisdom, and to learn their methods. As is the case for this book on Niguma yoga, our teachers offer technical details as they transmit their practices. We also learn how they have achieved their realizations. Then, as practitioners, we create our own personal fusion derived from our teachers, the teachings, and our own practice experience. While it is important to honor the lineage and maintain its integrity, we are not meant to be on automatic. We have to make the practice our own for optimal benefit. Still, careful observations of the trajectory of our teachers' lives, from their overarching path down to the most minute details, may offer valuable direction. We gain inspiration from a teacher's life story, their teachings, and the specific guidance they have given us to lift up our ordinary, daily lives. Each teacher can touch us in so many unique and different ways throughout our spiritual journey.

We may gain certain spiritual insights on the path from our human teachers. We may gain other insights from our direct experience of reality about such things as the nature of impermanence and the importance of making the most of the precious time we have available to achieve awakening. On the basis of teachings, life experience, and dedicated practice, various realizations may come to us at different stages. Those realizations may be immediate or gradual, or they may arise after long periods of concentrated practice, or we may receive guidance at one point but then realize its fruits much later.

For some, the benefit of study and practice comes instantly. That depends on our capacity and actually timing, and may be unrelated to whether one is intellectually bright or not. Sometimes students understand something instantly, and this leads them to think they are among the bright ones. However, the habit of self-aggrandizing warrants vigilance for it is something we should all avoid. To understand inner bliss and happiness, we must go beyond what goals we believe we have achieved. In spiritual pursuits, do not obsess over a short-term goal. The correct outlook is much more expansive through space and time; we should not practice only for immediate gratification. Rather we must be patient and take the long view, and when realizations arise, notice them but do not indulge. Similarly, when obstacles arise, take them in stride much the same way.

In my own case, I have had various teachers—some to learn specific practices, some for perspectives on my long-term spiritual journey, and those who have offered general guidance for my daily life. My first teacher, who recognized me as the incarnation of Kalu Rinpoche, was His Holiness Chatral Sangye Dorje Rinpoche. I have also been deeply influenced by Bokar Rinpoche, Tai Situ Rinpoche, and of course, most profoundly by His Holiness the Fourteenth Dalai Lama.

When I was first recognized as a Rinpoche, there was great expectation from the general public. The previous Kalu Rinpoche passed away in 1989. He was greatly revered by students all over the world and had left a profound legacy for the Shangpa lineage. I was born sixteen months later and was recognized in 1992. However, even when someone like me is recognized as a reincarnated teacher, it is still essential to study, practice, and aim to be skillful in daily life. Without this, being a Rinpoche in and of itself tends to be less fruitful. As a Buddhist practitioner, one has to practice in order to realize the fruits of the Dharma. In order to practice, one must receive proper instructions, learn the right techniques for the various teachings, and be exposed to the right example on which to model one's practice.

My first mentor, my spiritual father figure, was Bokar Rinpoche. He was a student of the previous Kalu Rinpoche. Bokar Rinpoche was quite close to his mentor and as a deeply dedicated student, he achieved profound realizations. Externally, Bokar Rinpoche appeared as a practitioner of all of the different traditions, just like previous Kalu Rinpoche. He practiced the Jonang tradition, the Kagyu tradition, the Dzogchen tradition, and the Kadam tradition of Gampopa. He practiced all of the different aspects of these traditions and showed respect and devotion to all of the great masters, especially to the previous Kalu Rinpoche. But his core practice was the five jewels of Niguma. I observed him practice the five jewels consistently during the years I spent with him. After my birth father passed away when I was seven, in 1997, Bokar Rinpoche became my primary spiritual mentor.

Traditionally, once you are recognized as a Rinpoche, you always sit on a throne during gatherings in the temple. Bokar Rinpoche removed the throne and told me that I had to live like a normal monk and learn a humble way of life. He wanted me to know the experience of simple monks and what they endure. He told me that if I was able to experience this, then I would be able to properly lead the monks and nuns. Otherwise, I wouldn't know the reality of how life is for them on a day-to-day basis, and I wouldn't be able to understand them, lead them, or earn respect from them. So, he removed the throne from the temple, and for a few years I did my monastic training alongside the other monks, starting with the study of vocal protocols for prayer and then moving on to learning to use traditional musical instruments.

For all these years, every day between 6:30 and 7:00 in the morning, I would go to Bokar Rinpoche's White Tara shrine room, prostrate to him three times, and say "Good morning." This is how I would start each day. Then I would go to the residential building and engage in my studies. Sometimes I was a lazy student—maybe most of the time. Even though I was very young then, between the ages of eleven and thirteen, Bokar Rinpoche was very compassionate to me, and very understanding. He was not forceful, but generous with his wisdom and skillful in his teaching methods. His explanations were clear and helpful. He spoke with me about how he saw the previous Kalu Rinpoche and how I should conduct myself as an incarnation of Kalu Rinpoche. At that time, I didn't fully recognize how great an enlightened being my predecessor was. Today, the more I practice over time, the more I feel that I am nothing compared to previous Kalu Rinpoche, especially with regard to his realizations. This is not a denial of myself as a reincarnation. More to the point, I am simply humbled by the great accomplishments of my predecessor.

There are points in time when a mentor is so kind as to give teachings and empowerments, but Bokar Rinpoche went above and beyond; he was kind enough to give me extensive teachings and empowerments that are part of an unbroken ear-to-ear lineage that the previous Kalu Rinpoche himself received, a tradition that stretches all the way back through history to Niguma. Rinpoche was incredibly generous with teachings, blessings, empowerments, and transmissions. Not only that, he actually built a retreat space for me. This is something you don't hear of very often, and I am forever grateful for that. All of this time with Bokar Rinpoche, I felt a deep heart connection and had complete trust in him.

During those several years I was with Bokar Rinpoche, he encouraged me to do extended retreat. From my point of view, you either do a traditional three-year retreat early in life or later in life, but usually not in between. When you do a retreat in the early stages of life, the mind becomes a little bit less diluted. You gain various insights in the way you perceive the Dharma, the way you receive teachings, and the way you practice. Then, when you do retreat later in life, it is much better because whatever life you had expected to lead, you have already gone through it—whether miserably or with success or somewhere in between. The only thing left for you to attempt to attain is a spiritual, Dharmic bliss. That is just my simple opinion; not everyone has to agree with me or follow my recommendation for when to do long retreat. But in between early and late life, when we are typically householders earning a livelihood, it is essential to work toward the benefit of all beings.

After receiving all the teachings, empowerments, and transmissions from Bokar Rinpoche, one year before his passing, I had a clairvoyant experience. At that time, I had a vision of a guardian protector of the Shangpa tradition named Kshitrapala while I was on the balcony struggling to memorize pages of scripture, something I had to do every day. At a certain stressful moment, this protector appeared to me and said, "You need to do a long life prayer for your abbot, and everyone has to do a long life prayer for him, too, not just in the monastery but throughout the region. We have to request all monasteries to participate." The protector then said, "This has to be done, otherwise there will be consequences."

As soon as I began to have this visitation from the protector, my entire experience of reality became a little bit blurry. Also, there was no actual spoken language used by either of us to communicate; we simply understood one another without uttering any words. As I sat there, I wondered who he was and who he represented. He said, "I am just a messenger of Six-Arm Mahakala." Six-Arm Mahakala is an emanation of Six-Arm Avalokiteshvara, also known as Chenrezig, who is a great compassionate being. I asked him if that was all, and he told me that that was the message in its entirety. After we concluded our brief conversation, the entire blurry reality of this vision absorbed and vanished. I then returned to a more solid reality in the way we typically perceive it. Soon after that, I went to see Bokar Rinpoche and told him the vision I had. His attendant and entourage were there; they looked at me like I was mentally unstable and like what I said was totally out of the blue, and just laughed. But when I delivered the message to Bokar Rinpoche, he gazed at me and expressed great appreciation. He received and welcomed the message. That was the moment that I understood definitively that Bokar Rinpoche was truly a realized being. With a beautiful glance, he said to me, "Rinpoche, I appreciate everything you experience, but when it is time to go, it is time to go." Later in my life, I recognized that this was a sign he was a realized being, because a realized being does not have fear of death. Rather, his focus is on the preciousness of life. That is the brief chapter of my experience and my journey with this mentor, Bokar Rinpoche.

If basic, virtuous qualities are not present and apparent, then whatever status may be attributed to an individual is irrelevant.

My second mentor and guide, who has served like my coach, is the Twelfth Tai Situ Rinpoche. Historically, there is thought to be a connection between Tai Situ Rinpoche and Kalu Rinpoche that has persisted over many lifetimes. However, history can be crafted over time by many different people—it can be presented from many different angles, depending on who benefits and how people want to portray themselves. Personally, I don't have any fantasies about the past. I can only simply say that we had a special relationship. My connection to and my appreciation and respect for Tai Situ Rinpoche developed in this lifetime. To the present day, it is an extraordinary bond between two human beings, not something borne of a fantasy that I hold from the past. If a great master cannot be a good, basic human being, whatever he or she claims to be is irrelevant. A priori, one must be a good, ordinary human being. If one has the qualities of honesty and courage to speak in black-and-white terms, knows when to speak and when not to speak, knows when to be decisive, and how to stand their ground, if they have basic human principles, then I can accept whatever they claim to be.

If basic, virtuous qualities are not present and apparent, then whatever status may be attributed to an individual is irrelevant. Many of us have seen images of the Buddha radiating golden light. In my view this is symbolic. My understanding is that a buddha does not radiate with rainbows and sun rays in people's eyes; a buddha radiates universal truth, and that truth magnifies their inner qualities naturally. It is spontaneous. We have to understand that great, realized beings do not hold that magical image, but simply hold and practice the universal truth, which we believe is the nature of the Buddhadharma.

Between Tai Situ Rinpoche and myself, our unique connection developed over a period of fifteen years. When I came out of my three-year retreat, I had no management skills, no understanding of what the reality of my responsibilities was going to look like. My mindset coming out of retreat may have been very pure, but it was not grounded in leadership experience. A pure mindset alone at a given point in time does not confer capacity to manage myriad expectations in a broad range of circumstances. Making a decision that is unpopular is not easy, but such action may be required if we are to be of true service. Tai Situ Rinpoche imparted this skill to me. He also gave me extensive Shangpa transmissions and encouraged me to lead Niguma teaching and practice. That was something I always wanted to do. Courage and support from a great realized being does not harm and only helps.

Tai Situ Rinpoche is not just the mentor who gave me the transmission of the Shangpa lineage; he also helped me understand that throughout history, humanity has always been beautiful and ugly at the same time, and it will remain that way for the foreseeable future. Just because we are disappointed with certain aspects of the world doesn't mean it will change. It will remain beautiful and ugly at the same time. People will do what is beneficial for themselves, either regardless of or at the expense of others. Some people will be greedy, while some will be deceitful and pretentious. It was Tai Situ Rinpoche who gave me the espresso-shot of reality to wake me up from my lazy morning. I am forever grateful for this great spiritual mentor. He is always kind and compassionate. He has told me, "If you are doing good, I will support you. If you are doing badly, it will be kind of difficult for me, but I will still support you." I'm so grateful for this inspiration, a fruit of his kindness.

Now I wish to share the enormous blessing of His Holiness the Fourteenth Dalai Lama. When you travel around the world establishing your own Dharma centers, sometimes you get caught up with dramas associated with center politics or the agendas of others. It can be difficult to maintain the deeper view of being a Buddhist practitioner. One may resort to a more narrow and limited mindset: How should we renovate this Dharma center? How should we raise funds for that monastery? How can we clean up the debt? How do we execute this project? There are piles of never-ending crises that need handling. It is easy to forget who you are in these moments and lose sight of certain aspects of the Dharma.

Listening to the teachings of His Holiness the Dalai Lama around the world, one gains a wider perspective of what it means to be a practitioner and the importance of making a broad, positive impact on this world. He is not on a quest to convert others, nor does he speak from a specifically religious platform. Rather, his teachings free people from blind faith and help ensure that they are focused on the practical effort to bring greater happiness to humanity. That has been the activity of His Holiness the Dalai Lama for many decades. There is great benefit in receiving his teachings and observing his methods in their stark simplicity. These teachings have given me an important understanding of what the world actually needs. His Holiness the Dalai Lama has the knowledge of every deeply profound Buddhist teaching, and yet he chooses to focus his practice on Avalokiteshvara, who embodies loving-kindness, compassion, and meditation, and in this way he brings a great happiness to humanity. This is not because he doesn't know enough—he knows everything, but he sees the capacity that each of us has as human beings, and he understands that many simply hold blind faith, which is by nature a fixed view. Buddhist practitioners are not immune to this pitfall, and this leads to a lot of conflict between religions and nations.

Blind faith has a negative ripple effect on our global harmony. That is why His Holiness doesn't promote Buddhism first. Instead, he promotes loving-kindness first. Then he promotes meditation and compassion. This is because he understands what is most needed by the world.

In my own personal experience as a Dharma practitioner, I've found that if we try to practice all of the empowerments we have received, it is impossible to finish in a day, even in a lifetime. Second, at this point in the history of human civilization, our minds tend to become distracted, weakened, and diluted. We are more exposed to pollution, microplastics, and toxic mentalities. But planetary challenges come down to our human behavior. If we can provide a little bit of spiritual understanding to ease and cool down the sometimes hot and aggressive nature of human behavior, that is a great contribution to the human world and our society. It is in this vein that I wish to teach Niguma yoga. At its foundation, this is a powerful practice for physical and mental well-being. This is where my inspiration comes from. Remember once more, Niguma Yoga is a practice that can be done by virtually anyone.

I have just discussed my three principal mentors because they are very special to me. They have been incredibly kind to me and a source of blessings. Therefore, it is important to mention them before I proceed with the subject of practicing the yoga of Niguma. However, in understanding my role, please know that in the context of Niguma yoga, there is no need to see me as a guru. For you I simply wish to be a guide, as you cultivate your own spiritual life.

ORGANIZATION OF THE BOOK

The first chapter discusses the lineage of these practices of Niguma and how they eventually came to us. The second chapter covers guidance on the preparation of the mind and body for the practice, including a discussion on the foundation of meditation, guidance on maintaining emotional balance, and the correct mental attitude with which to approach the yoga of Niguma. Chapter three shares traditional yogic lifestyle recommendations and health considerations before and during your practice and is cowritten with Michele Loew based on her many years of experience with hatha yoga and Ayurvedic medicine, and her interest in the sister science of Sowa Rigpa, Tibetan medicine. The fourth chapter on building your Niguma practice teaches the foundational postures used throughout the practice, including how I teach vase breathing. Additionally, Michele offers guidance on basic breathing techniques that will provide you awareness into how to effectively work with diaphragmatic breathing for your overall health, which also prepares you for breathing correctly in the yoga of Niguma. Chapter five presents the actual sequence of postures of the yoga of Niguma with sketches and descriptions, as well as guidance from Michele on practices from hatha yoga that will support and prepare the body to practice this form. In chapter six I give some final words of encouragement for you to commit to your practice, give homage to the Buddha's teachings, and speak on the importance of maintaining the pristine path of Niguma's lineage. Finally, there is an appendix Michele has designed for you containing important preliminary stretches you can use to open your hips and body, with our hopes of making the yoga of Niguma more accessible to you.

More support for your Niguma yoga practice is available to you online. We have created video resources for you to supplement the teachings in this book. You can access those online at:

www.wisdomexperience.org/niguma-yoga-poses-kalu-rinpoche.

Part 1
Introducing Niguma Yoga

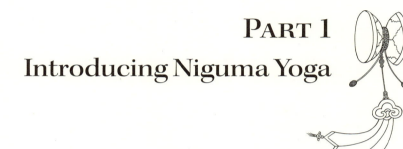

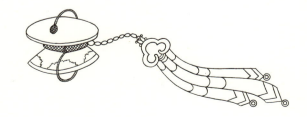

1

The Lineage of the Practices

THE HISTORY OF NIGUMA AND HER RELEVANCE TO US

In the Vajrayana tradition it is essential to take stock of one's spiritual heritage by understanding the roots of the lineage and its trajectory over time. Niguma was an Indian mahasiddha who lived approximately a thousand years ago in what is now Kashmir, located in the northern part of the country. A *mahasiddha* is a great realized being. There were many mahasiddhas in India, but Niguma was a tenth-level bodhisattva, which is equivalent to Tara and Avalokiteshvara. Niguma herself was a student of many other great mahasiddhas. She was born into the Brahmin caste, which is the highest social class. She was related to Naropa, one of the great Buddhist yogis of his time. Some sources say that Naropa was her elder brother, others that Naropa was her cousin or relative—so the nature of their relationship depends on which book you read. It doesn't matter, though, because it doesn't impact the teachings or the Niguma yoga we are to do.

Niguma practiced for many years while living the simple life of a yogini. Today, some think of a yogi or yogini as a person who goes a little over the top or crazy. Niguma did not live through the eyes of others. She was an individual and made no distinction between those who criticized her and those who praised her. She made no distinction between those with a pile of sand or a pile of gold. She lived a very ascetic life in the forest, far away from the busy world. From time to time, she met with other practitioners like herself. Niguma once made a statement that she had no guru or mentor other than the Buddha himself. This was not to boast. Rather, it demonstrated her level of realization. She left an extensive and profound legacy of teachings that was instrumental in bringing Vajrayana Dharma from India into the Himalayan region and beyond. Her principal contributions lie in the methods she imparted to practitioners to realize the illusory nature of existence. Realizing this illusory nature, as distinct from a fixed view, allows the myriad delusions of body, speech, and mind to soften and finally fall away. Unless and until illusory nature is realized, we remain slaves to our coarse and subtle emotions, which at their foundation consist of ignorance, aversion, and attachment, and then, like the color palette of an artist, granulate into jealousy, fear, sadness, resentment, anxiety, pride, habituation, and so on. Illusory nature is the portal to liberation because once it softens the ordinary, solid, false view of self, then the objects we behold and judge ultimately cease to exist in the same way. This is the practice of freedom.

The actual yoga of Niguma is foundational to the realization of illusory nature insofar as it clears and strengthens the subtle energetic channels within the body, fortifies the gross physical form, and ultimately prepares the mindstream to take up the profound meditation practices that then follow, resulting in full awakening.

Niguma's teachings were brought to Tibet by Khyungpo Naljor. He was a Bon practitioner until his mid-fifties, then he became a Kadam practitioner and a Dzogchen practitioner. Bon is the spiritual tradition that existed prior to the arrival of the Dharma in the Himalayan region. The Kadam practitioners engaged in a series of analytical meditations, described as the graduated path, and Dzogchen is the practice of emptiness. After that he traveled to Nepal and then to Bodh Gaya in India. When he reached Bodh Gaya, Khyungpo Naljor met Dorje Denpa, the abbot of the Mahabodhi Temple. It was there that he was introduced to the name of Niguma; he was inspired upon hearing of this female yogi who was residing in a very fearful charnel ground, a place where corpses are taken. So he went there to look for Niguma, and after making earnest prayers, finally met her. The first time he made prostrations to her and requested teachings, she responded saying, "I am a cannibal. I am going to come back with my friends and we are going to eat you alive." Obviously, if I were in that situation, I would probably take the suggestion and leave instantly. I would also stop walking around the forest seeking a spiritual awakening. But Khyungpo Naljor was not deterred. He decided to stick around. You have to keep in mind that he was not just some random dude; he was already an advanced practitioner praised by other great masters. So he had an instinct to stick with it. He then offered Niguma gold dust. She picked up the gold dust and thrust it away into the forest. She then asked Khyungpo Naljor, "What do you think of that? Do you think there is a golden river, golden mountains, and golden forest?" Khyungpo Naljor replied, "No. That is your manifestation. That is you performing miracles."

Niguma replied, "If you have a pure mind, everywhere and anywhere is a pure land. If you have an impure mind, everywhere and anywhere is an impure land, and there is no escaping it." Whether she performed a miracle with the gold dust is not the important message here. The important message is looking at how we receive the teachings and how practice can change our perceptions of life. Niguma then gave Khyungpo Naljor complete teachings on the six yogas of Niguma as well as the five golden Dharmas of Niguma. These are very special teachings that were revered, studied, and practiced by Niguma practitioners and all major and smaller branches of Vajrayana Buddhism—including Drukpa Kagyu, Sakya, Gelug, and Jonang practitioners. The yoga of Niguma, which we are practicing in this book, is associated with the breathing practice that is the first of the six yogas of Niguma; the remainder are illusory body, dream yoga, luminosity, the transference of consciousness (*phowa*), and the intermediate state after death (*bardo*).

Eventually, Niguma gave the full transmission to Khyungpo Naljor while he was in a state of lucid dreaming. She told him that neither he nor future practitioners were allowed to share these teachings, other than ear-to-ear to one student each generation, until the seventh generation, beginning with Niguma herself. After the seventh generation, the teachings of Niguma could be shared but still carefully guarded. Gradually these Shangpa traditions were shared with all of the various Vajrayana traditions over the past thousand years, and are now practiced widely among Vajrayana practitioners.

Niguma's teachings and practices are connected to my life through the previous Kalu Rinpoche. He was one of the principal practitioners who revived the Shangpa lineage. Strict secrecy was kept during the first seven generations of practitioners and the teachings were held with careful discretion thereafter, which served to keep the lineage pure, but also limited access. That is the tradeoff. So, there was limited transmission, continuing discretion plus secrecy, and geopolitical changes with their associated regional instability. These factors were responsible for the Shangpa Kagyu tradition ending up as one of minor linages, not because it was less important but because it was smaller. As Kalu Rinpoche's reincarnation, I carry on his teachings and work to maintain his legacy, including the tradition of the three-year retreat. However, in order for you to realize the benefit to body and mind of imbibing the essence of the tradition, I made the decision to write this book. This is an unprecedented gesture to create broad access to Niguma yoga for Buddhists and non-Buddhists alike and particularly for the millions of hatha yoga practitioners. My wish is that through this practice, you become physically well and mentally resilient, and can travel along the journey toward clarity and awakening.

Part 2

Preparation of Mind and Body and Practical Guidance for the Yogic Lifestyle

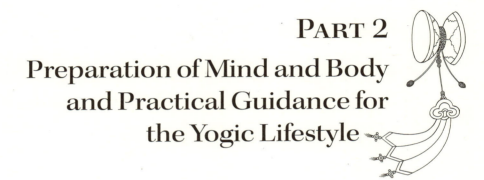

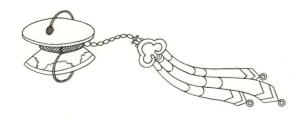

2

Preparation of the Mind

Lacking awareness of our own emotions and of our own ego is just like living under the same roof as a thief.

The yoga of Niguma is open to you regardless of your faith background or spiritual understanding. That is because each of us is breathing, and each of us has a sense of awareness, clarity, and calmness in our mind. Regardless of where we were born or to which cultures we have become accustomed, we all seek happiness. We also wish for deep contentment that reaches down into our subconscious state of mind. Furthermore, we want to be joyful, and we want to share that experience of joy with those whom we dearly love. It is therefore highly important to cultivate a sense of clarity of mind and to develop resilience combined with wisdom. In order to reach this level of understanding, so much depends on clarity in our relationship to sensory inputs: vision, hearing, taste, touch, smell, and mentation. These six senses are neither inherently positive nor negative. However, when we lack an understanding that these are merely sense windows, we may be subject to deceptive states, such as pride. Still, even pride itself is not inherently negative or positive. Ordinary pride is simply the reflection of one's own illusory ego, but there is also divine pride, free of ego.

However, even when the ego is present, it does not mean that you are a bad person. Anyone can point to another person and claim that they have a big ego. Who really knows if any given individual can spot another person's ego and accurately paint such a label on them?

Let's not divert our attention to such considerations. Rather, let's dedicate our efforts and capacity toward reaching a state of clarity. Time is short, and we are very vulnerable, more vulnerable than we think we are. We are vulnerable to external and internal threats, including people, animals, disease, and climate. We are even more vulnerable to our own emotions. Lacking awareness of our own emotions and of our own ego is just like living under the same roof as a thief.

We each have a vital responsibility to develop universal understanding in order to contribute to a harmonious world in the vastness of time and space and in the intimacy of the moment with those we love and our community. Almost without exception, we say that we want to love the world and that we must take care of one another. We then engage in efforts of service and charity. However, to do so skillfully, it is essential that, through awareness, we find harmony within, especially with regard to our emotions.

This can be very difficult. A person who says "I have no ego" definitely has an ego. A person who says "I have no jealousy" definitely has jealousy. But the existence of jealousy reflects an attachment to self; it has nothing to do with others. Quelling emotions requires a sense of awareness of our own emotions and action. Mindful action can only occur in each moment, and it may not be helpful to automatically restrict ourselves to a fixed set of behavioral guidelines. It is also important to bear in mind that we should not blindly force ourselves into a deluded sense of service. There is no justification to punish yourself for the greater good. Right action must uplift each person in the journey of spiritual awakening, including oneself.

Meditation and yoga are key methods to cultivate mindful and effective action. The reason I teach Niguma yoga is that it can be beneficial without regard to any specific faith or religion. At their origins, all faiths have a beautiful simplicity and speak of a fundamental human connection. However, following the genesis of a given faith, institutions may develop, and power struggles or political factions may arise. In such cases, it is important to focus on our own personal challenges, which stem from our ego and resultant pride, and the delusions that then arise, which trigger our emotions and shape our actions. We should look within for insights rather than focusing on all the external matters that arise.

As such, it is essential to look after one's body and mind. This is true no matter one's age. Some people say, "I am young and therefore don't need to look after my body. I can do all sorts of different experiments, get intoxicated, and misbehave all I want." But that creates all sorts of disharmony that lasts throughout one's lifetime. Why do that? Then there are those who consider themselves "old people," and for this reason never engage in actions that may benefit body and mind. Both of these views are wrong and therefore, regardless of our age, we must focus on our core purpose, which is to develop inner harmony. Once we cultivate inner harmony, our daily activities will bring benefit to all sentient beings. When there is genuine inner harmony, it is no longer necessary to take up heroic efforts or complicated doctrines to remind us what need to do and what we should say, think, and so on.

Therefore, I want to introduce to you Niguma yoga, which includes a sequence of twenty-five physical sets of actions. Usually, when this is taught in a Buddhist context, a practitioner will take up traditional teachings and put them into practice. The teachings of Niguma are very beautiful, very simple, and very profound, while also being readily understandable. These attributes reflect the wisdom of the teachings.

To be clear, the yoga of Niguma, or Niguma yoga, is different than the *yogas* of Niguma. The latter refers to the six yogas of Niguma, which are, to reiterate, tummo breathing meditation, illusory body, dream yoga, luminosity, transference of consciousness, and bardo, which here primarily refers to the intermediate state between death and rebirth. The yoga of Niguma is the topic of this book, and if studied in the context of the six yogas of Niguma, is done in conjunction with the first yoga, which is tummo. To be clear, Niguma yoga magnifies the effect of tummo and not the other way around. So, the yoga of Niguma is not among the six yogas of Niguma but it is advisable to couple tummo, the first yoga, with the yoga of Niguma,

The yoga of Niguma consists of twenty-five sets of physical postures that have a strong relationship to spiritual and energetic phenomena. Because tummo is more delicate and more challenging, it is not within the scope of this book, and I have reserved instruction on this practice for in-person gatherings. Please also bear in mind that while tummo, if properly transmitted, can be done by itself, the yoga of Niguma may be unsafe unless the practitioner maintains a solid, isometric core and manages the breath appropriately.

The wisdom of Niguma, a great enlightened being, is widely accessible. Even at eighty years old, it is possible to take up the teachings, and even then the yoga practice can be adapted to suit your physicality. With regard to the younger generations, the teachings of Niguma are not based on blind faith or adherence to a specific culture, but rather focused on developing physical health, mental well-being, calm abiding, and resilience. In this way, Niguma yoga is introduced such that anyone can take up the practice. You do not need a guru. You do not need me. You do not need mystical objects or beliefs. All you need is your breath, your awareness, and your physical action. The path of Niguma yoga involves integrating your body, your mind, and your breath.

Niguma was a great enlightened female being, though it should be understood there is no difference between female and male practitioners. There is no gender prejudice or discrimination with regard to who has the capacity for realization from the practice.

CALM ABIDING: THE FOUNDATION OF MEDITATION

When it comes to meditation, people often have a misconception that to meditate is to think of nothing. That, in fact, is not the right understanding of calm-abiding meditation, known as *shamatha* in Sanskrit. Another common misconception is the idea that meditation is like being on a "trip." Simply disconnecting from reality through the imagination is also not meditation, regardless of how beautiful the imagination might be. Calm-abiding meditation involves maintaining the pristine presence of awareness without a fixed focus on any external object. One remains uninvolved with whatever arises by simply noticing it and letting it pass away, then returning one's attention to the breath. It requires three elements: First, clarity to detect gross and subtle distraction. Second, to remain in a refined, fluid, nongrasping state of mind, rather than becoming lost in objects that transiently arise. Finally, it requires an understanding that the very essence of meditation is emptiness held with clarity, calmness, and transparency, while still always maintaining concentration to detect distraction—whether ordinary or subtle—allowing it to fall away and then returning to the breath.

Many traditions have cultivated meditation techniques since the time of the Buddha, utilizing myriad methods throughout history, but there is one current approach to meditation in which people like to make up things on their own, without a sense of history or method. Be aware that this can lead to a dangerous conclusions. Anytime you consider working with a new teacher or practice it is essential that you check up, do your homework, and confirm for yourself that the method comes from an authentic meditation tradition and that the teacher is accomplished and ethical. Then, the correct method for learning calm abiding starts with a breathing exercise. Object-based approaches can be difficult, because they can carry a burden of concentration on the object. The easier way is to base the attention on one's breathing. Many meditators like to count twenty-one breaths without distraction, but I would recommend avoiding counting the breaths and instead focus on riding the rhythm of the breath with the mind. Focus on the experience of the breath going through the nose without considering where the air is coming from and where it is going. Keep the mind on the sensation of the breath, free of judgment about how, when, and where.

When you sense a state of calmness, recognize that everything is bound to change and is impermanent. Always just come back to the breath, and know that we are all the same in this way. Keep returning to the breath. Consider that all sentient beings want to be free from suffering, and that we are all the same in this way, and then again come back to the breath. When you come back for the third round, wish for all sentient beings to find the joy that you have found, and then visualize them with the radiance of positivity.

Once again, remember that, first, everything is bound to change and all phenomena are of the nature of impermanence. Second, all sentient beings do not wish to suffer and seek happiness, so we are all the same. Third, dedicate each meditation to all sentient beings such that they can experience the radiance of calm abiding and share it with others.

MENTAL ATTITUDE: FINDING THE BALANCE IN OUR EMOTIONS AND THE PRACTICE

Our attitude toward life changes throughout the various stages of our development. It is no different than the evolution of our spiritual journey. The foundation doesn't change, but how you see it, how calmly you see it, how profoundly you see it, how you maintain your attitude throughout the day and night—these phenomena become refined over time. The foundation doesn't change one's mental attitude, but the whole experience is one of gradual refinement. To be short and clear, it doesn't stay the same. For example, our perspective on life when we are a child or a teenager is more formative. The scope and depth of what we see tends to be more limited, given that our experience and knowledge is at an early stage of development.

As we evolve over time, for most, life becomes more meaningful and fruitful. Others may just be waiting to die. Life becomes very monotonous, and some people hope to be picked up by a higher power and carried away rather than living fully throughout their lifetime. In Niguma yoga, our foundational mental attitude doesn't change. However, as we practice, our mental attitude moves into an expansion of calmness. In contrast to the typical human pattern of overthinking, for some, a profound mental calmness gradually arises. Such outcomes depend on how well one maintains their Niguma yoga practice and whether one recognizes their gross and subtle distractions, and a host of other elements.

What is our mental attitude in Niguma yoga? In my personal experience, it is really simple, but how you feel within your body and mind changes, and there is an immense experience of clarity, joy, and calm contentment as you progress with the practice. For me, it started by experiencing calm and quiet, and eventually reached the point where I could say, "Everything is fine. Everything is good. Even if I die right now, still everything is good. I expect nothing less and nothing more." You can go into that gentle mental attitude throughout your practice.

You may start your practice of Niguma yoga with thoughts like: "I need to be calm. I need to focus. I need to be careful. I need to execute the correct physical movements. I cannot do it wrong. I need to exhale and inhale, breathe at the right pace and time." We get into this self-micromanaging attitude. But as you progress in your practice, don't think that this is wrong. It is simply how you start. Over time, as you practice, the calmness and experience of the vastness of the mind will come all by itself. That very experience relieves any sense of vulnerability or expectation. At the same time, you begin to recognize the vastness of your mindset, like looking out over space. With that sort of mindset, that sort of capacity, you see your progress. The practice is not a problem to be solved but a mystery to be lived; it is an experience you are able to live in. As you progress in your practice, you will also be able to feel the blood and energy flow within the body. This happens naturally, all by itself, without overthinking it. If you overthink, saying, "I have good energy" or "I have bad energy," in that moment, you are not on the right track. Don't take up such expectations that you need to feel this or that energy. None of that should be a priority. Also, it helps to simply refrain from naming an experience or sensation. Instead, just allow phenomena to arise and pass away without a name. By naming, we give a phenomenon a misguided sense of solid existence. Just do the practice, and over time the positive fruits will arise, and you will feel incredible mental and physical resilience and continuous awareness.

To develop your mental attitude and spiritual qualities with this yoga practice, your first step is to accept impermanence. There is no need to experience despair or sadness in the face of change. All positive and negative emotions simply arise, and at some point, pass away.

> *Everything that has a beginning has an end, everything that is happening right now is constantly changing, and everything is impermanent and bound to change—and will change.*

Think of impermanence as constant change. Everything is bound to change. Everything that has a beginning has an end. Hearing just one sentence about impermanence may be enough for you to let go of some fixation in your mind. Over time, progressively, an understanding of the meaning of impermanence will come by itself. There are three things to accept: everything that has a beginning has an end, everything that is happening right now is constantly changing, and everything is impermanent and bound to change—and will change. By keeping these acceptances in mind, you minimize the illusion of your ego. When you minimize the illusion of your ego, you give fewer resources to your fixation. When you give fewer resources to your fixation, the truth will no longer be elusive, but right in front of you. At that time the blissful journey will open up for you. So, don't worry about it if you don't have a heart-rending understanding of impermanence. Keep your expectation low when it comes to the realization of impermanence. Just keep it simple with these three principals: Everything is bound to change. Everything that has a beginning has an end. Everything is constantly changing. As long as you try to accept that or try to chant it like a mantra in your mind, the fixation will dissolve over time by itself. That is the first step.

The second step, when you are doing the yoga sequence, is to refrain from thinking that you are starting something that you have to complete. Don't think, "I have to finish this. I have to repeat the poses so many times." All of that has to be abandoned. There is no such thing as "finishing" it. Just like your ego and the illusion of jealousy have no end, your practice has no end. Eventually, the fruit of the practice will overwhelm your negativity. Therefore, abandon thoughts of how many times you have done the practice, how long you have done it, or when are you going to finish it. Then you will be able to more clearly experience the sensation of the breath, the sensation of the body, and the sensation of the mind.

The final point about mental attitudes during the practice of Niguma yoga is that after one sequence, you should not rush into the next. Don't think, "What is my next posture? When do I breathe in?" Don't think ahead. Keep the sequence at a medium pace with a normal heart rate. Don't over-prepare. Just be gentle with yourself. It is important that you don't forget to be gentle—so many spiritual seekers these days are harsh on themselves. But being harsh won't get you anywhere. Being gentle and not exhausting yourself are important keys to succeed in this practice. Therefore, when you are engaged in the yoga, in between sequences, don't think, "Now I've finished the first sequence, now I am moving to the second sequence." If you have a thought like, "Now, I want to repeat the third sequence maybe two more times, " do it, but do it gently. Always keep your body, mind, and breath as a unity.

Always keep your body, mind, and breath as a unity.

Balancing Emotions and Daily Activities with the Practice

Let's go over how to balance your emotions and everyday activities with Niguma yoga. I will keep it very simple. If you take away anything from this material, keep the following in mind: Don't take on the idea that you want to apply this practice to your daily life. Expectations like that are nonsense that we try to feed ourselves, and should be avoided as much as possible. What happens is that whenever you have an expectation, you set yourself up for disappointment. The fixed goal itself can be an obstacle to experiencing things as they truly are in each moment as they arise. Of course, if you don't practice appropriately, you cannot bring it into your life. But you can't force it. If you practice genuinely, sincerely, and honestly from the bottom of your heart, it can influence your behavior, your decisions, your perception of reality, and how you react to things. However, if you *try* to bring the practice into your life, into your decision making, or into your struggle with emotions, you will fail miserably because the practice is not a fungible token that you can redeem. Many people think that bringing the practice into daily life is like using a coupon at the store. We think that we can use one coupon today and another one tomorrow. It doesn't work like that, however, because our mental attitude must develop first. Without clarity and calmness in our mind, the thought of bringing the yoga into your life is simply an overestimation of your capacity. It is simple: just practice, and the positivity will come all by itself.

Opening the flower of positivity can be can be elusive.

Take a look at anger, for example. Say you have an argument with a person, and now your entire day is ruined. You can see the effect negativity has on your life. So many of us accept that, but opening the flower of positivity can be elusive. There is a common misconception that somehow the fruits of Niguma yoga practice are transactional. We would like to collect the resulting merit of the practice in the manner and timeframe we desire. Yet the fruits of the practice are not merchantable. The practice has to be part of your habit, part of your routine. Then it will influence your decision making and your perception of reality, because the decision comes down to how you perceive your reality. It depends on how calm you are. How we perceive reality depends upon our ability to see beyond the illusion of our mind. If we see beyond the illusion of anger and jealousy, then we have far greater insight. The clearer your understanding of how your emotions function, the greater the insight. The greater the insight, the more meaningful and conclusive the decisions you make will be, whether about a family or business matter or life in general.

Additionally, as yoga practitioners, we need to be aware of the food we consume, because what we consume has an effect on the chemicals in our brain and body as well as how our body and mind react and function. In turn, this has an effect on how we can practice and how physically active we can be. The body and mind have to work together. Some people may think that because they are so spiritual, they don't need to care about what they eat. I am not here to promote being a vegetarian or vegan or any particular diet. But we can glean insight from the relationship monks had with food during the time of Buddha, when they'd fast a little bit after midday, only consuming what was needed for the body; for us, too, being aware of what we consume is important. Balanced nutrition not based on sugars and starches but with more whole grain causes our body to be more balanced. If you consume what is harmonious for your body and at the time and in the amount that suits your body, you will find it easier to remain in emotional and physical balance. The mind is more calm and clear.

With regard to intoxicants, it goes without saying that the mind is more calm and clear when one avoids the consumption of alcohol and tobacco. This is also the case, for any other pharmaceutical or street drugs that dull or numb the system, drain our energy, or result in habituation. There are also two schools of thought with regard to the vow to refrain from intoxicants: The first view is simply zero tolerance. It holds that any intoxicants are harmful. Perhaps a small amount is less harmful, but intoxicants are to be strictly avoided. The second view is that some agents taken in moderation, such that one does not lose control, are acceptable. Having said this, there is always a tendency, large or small, to roll down the slippery slope. Many times people think that they will have only one drink but that drink makes them believe they are fine to keep going.

Finally, I ask you to be aware that whenever you read these teachings or practice the yoga of Niguma, you should not assume that you know everything. Otherwise, you risk creating your own obstacles. Instead, keep yourself humble, gentle, and clearheaded. But know that being humble does not mean letting people walk over you in daily life.

Whenever you read texts from the Buddha or from other masters or scholars, the guidance is to keep a humble and open attitude of not-knowing. Having that sense of openness is important. And in all our traditions, having universal respect is vital.

Knowing your own limitations is also important. Practice what you can commit to, and what you are able to handle. Many people receive teachings about a lot of practices, but their progress in those practices is limited because they have such a large number of commitments. If you have a question about how to engage in the various teachings you've received, you may wish to seek the advice of your mentors. You may get different answers, though, and they may conflict. That can pose its own challenge, but it's worth the effort. In balance, as we have said before, blind faith can be dangerous. As much as you may respect the teachings and your teachers, you must always make your own choices from among all the guidance you receive. That may include choosing to engage in something you may not fully understand because of a sense of trust. It may sound like I just made two contradictory statements. If so, think about it.

3

Yogic Lifestyle: Health, Safety, and Practical Guidance

Before beginning physical yoga and breathing practices, it is important to check in with your overall health and make any changes that will ensure the practice is beneficial and safe. This chapter gives some practical suggestions on yogic lifestyle and preliminaries that I hope you will consider so this practice can be optimally supportive to your well-being.

Guidance on Physical Health

Traditionally, a yoga student would consult with their close guru or yogic master to receive guidance on any dietary changes or cleansing preparations for internal health before starting a serious practice. Today, a check-up with a healthcare professional who knows you and can guide your optimal health with good modern diagnostics and recommendations is a great support on the path. Consider having periodic physical exams to make sure you are caring for your body in the best way possible so your practice will serve your highest good and create no harm. If you have preexisting health issues, please get approval from your doctor before practicing. Let the doctor know that this type of yoga utilizes breath retentions, and that some of the sequences require standing up and sitting down from the ground to build leg strength and stamina. Let them know this practice is less about stretching and more about building energy; cardiovascular health; respiratory fitness; strengthening muscles, bones, and joints; increased adrenaline; lung capacity; brain health; and a strong core. If you have weaknesses in those areas, your doctor might want you to avoid the practice altogether, or they might have you focus on the gentler sequences, preliminary stretches, and preparatory breathing practices that are shared in this book, as they are generally accessible to most and extremely beneficial for recovering health. Have a conversation with your health care provider, perhaps even consider sharing this book with them, and determine which exercises will be most supportive and kind to your body in its current condition. Be encouraged that even a little practice will bring you progress on your path to greater health. Also consider finding an opportunity to practice with us in person so we can personally guide you.

APPROACHING THE PHYSICAL PRACTICE INTELLIGENTLY

When beginning to train, you don't have to do all twenty-five Niguma yoga exercises consecutively. There are some sequences that are gentler and some that will take more preparation, training, physical fitness, and stamina to be ready for. If you are healthy but completely new to physical yoga practice, be patient and practice slowly. With continued practice of even a few sequences daily, you will increase your breathing capacity and cardiovascular health and find ease in building up to the full series. We give modifications and adaptations you can try, but if you find yourself struggling in a sequence, do more preparations and work with the postures that are available to you now.

Even seasoned hatha yoga practitioners will at first find the breath retentions and simultaneous physical movements a new challenge. Meet yourself where you are at and build compassion for yourself so you can truly give it to others. It takes time, consistent practice, and patience to reach a place of effortlessness and ease. Pushing too hard and striving can not only damage your body but keep you from reaching higher states of awareness and bliss. If you find yourself too out of breath or your heart rate feels high, consider focusing on the seated sequences from sequences 18 to 23 first. These are much less difficult and very calming to the nervous system.

Sequences 1 to 13 and 24 to 25 are more demanding physically, increase adrenaline, and build stamina and the cardiovascular system. They are ultimately a great boon to our overall health and longevity. Nevertheless, beginners can feel winded and should practice patience by adding on only a few sequences at a time.

Take pause after each sequence to connect to your physical body and sense how you feel. Becoming intimate with your body, its sensations, and the pace and flow of breath is an important part of growing your yoga practice.

Sequences 14 to 17 focus on the subtle body energy purification, so check in with how your nervous system feels after practicing and be aware of the emotional body and acknowledge any increased emotional sensitivity.

Find a support system of loving friends, community, a spiritual mentor, and/ or a therapist who can give you guidance and any needed care as you release and cleanse the emotional body.

GUIDANCE ON MENTAL HEALTH AND WIND IMBALANCES

If you have a history of mental illness, you must get approval and support from your mental health care provider before beginning yoga practice. Having a balanced state of mind is a prerequisite for starting out on this transformational journey to absolute happiness. Tibetan medicine, Sowa Rigpa, and its sister science, Indian Ayurvedic medicine, have done a great deal of research studying wind-related mental illness, what is called *sog lung trugpa* (Tib. སོག་རླུང་འཁྲུག་པ་) in Tibetan medicine, or *vata* disturbance in Ayurveda. Western researchers are also beginning to study wind-related diagnoses in mental health, such as the 2019 National Institute of Health study "rLung, Mind, and Mental Health: The Notion of 'Wind' in Tibetan Conceptions of Mind and Mental Illness."

When wind becomes too high or disturbed from blockages in the mind and subtle body, it can negatively affect the body and mind. This is why going slowly, staying grounded, eating nutritious foods, sleeping well, staying warm, finding support to stay calm, and avoiding intoxicants is so important when engaging in transformative yoga practices such as the yoga of Niguma. If, after commencing a daily yoga practice, you have an increase of any of the following symptoms, please stop performing the sequences and the breath retentions, seek support, and ground yourself. I have listed some supportive traditional remedies below.

The following are symptoms of a wind (*sog lung*) disorder:

- Disturbed sleep
- Excessive yawning
- Anxiety
- Heavy, tight chest and/or shortness of breath
- Increased blood pressure
- Abnormal all-over joint pain
- Lack of appetite
- Spaciness
- Vertigo
- Excessive talking
- Irritability and uncontrollable emotions
- Headaches
- Struggling with concentration
- Dizziness
- Common anxiety or depression symptoms

The following are traditional supportive remedies from Tibetan and Ayurvedic medicine used to calm the winds:

- Calm-abiding meditation
- Spending time in nature
- Slow walks
- Receiving warm-oil or hot-stone massage

- Acupuncture or Tibetan moxibustion
- Soaking in warm mineral baths
- Eating warm, oily foods
- Sleep meditation practices and getting good sleep
- Restorative yoga
- Butter tea and ghee
- Warm tea, nutmeg, and warm milk
- Bone broth or vegetable broth with spices like ginger, turmeric, rosemary, cloves, and peppers to warm the body
- Detoxing from news and social media
- Listening to calming music or singing bowls

LIFESTYLE OF A YOGI

As a householder with a busy life, you must be realistic about how much you can take on. Remember, even a little practice helps, and the last thing you want to do is create more stress from unmeetable demands. We are not living in the time of Niguma, in the forest, or on retreat. But if you practice with sincerity and with heartfelt motivation, little by little you will find yourself making more time for this practice until it genuinely affects every aspect of your life positively. Eventually, you might practice with the same motivation as the great yogis of the time of Niguma. And in turn, all aspects of life become the practice. How you eat, sleep, and connect in relationship all become important and seeped with wisdom and compassion. You see your life as precious and see having a healthy, long life as an opportunity to practice and serve others. Make a commitment to do what you can now, and as your practice evolves, you will find that you may become more interested in caring for yourself in that light. Treatises on yoga by the mahasiddhas, the great adepts of Vajrayana and hatha yoga who lived at the time of Niguma and onward, also stress the importance of the body being healthy and free from illness and the mind being stable prior to beginning physical yoga. This was part of the spiritual path, and it also served to prepare the body and mind for the powerful movement of subtle body energy freely into the central channel, awakening enlightened mind. They also gave techniques to reduce inflammation, which was considered to be harmful even in ancient times. The *Hatha Pradipika*, which became a template for classical hatha yoga, was a compilation of yoga practices passed on from the oral traditions and put into writing by Svatmarama in the 1450s. It emphasizes preliminary cleansing techniques and dietary recommendations that are required to be performed prior to beginning breath work and yoga poses to protect the yogi from mental obscurations and subtle body blockages, which could result in the subtle body wind disturbances we have listed above. It gives a list of foods that are harmful to a yogi and also lists beneficial foods, similar to what we have shared. Then it covers detailed breathing to reduce inflammation and finally breath retention and yoga postures to support progressively reaching the high pinnacle of raja yoga, samadhi. It stresses, as does the yoga of Niguma and Vajrayana Buddhism, that our vital subtle body energy (*prana*) and our mind (*chitta*) are inseparable, and thus we must attend to them both. In this same way, keep in mind the importance of shifting gradually toward more mindfulness in all aspects of your life, until eating, breathing, sleeping, and physical movements are all part of your spiritual daily practice. But again, this will happen as an outpouring of your daily practice. You don't have to set unrealistic goals. Just try to show up each day in some way to practice.

The Breath and Sleep

Today, modern scientific research is validating the wisdom of these early yogic traditions with clinical studies showing how harmful poor diet, stress, incorrect breathing, and lack of sleep are to our physical and mental well-being. These all create inflammation and early aging. If we truly want to be of benefit to all sentient beings, we must practice on and off our yoga cushion, doing the best we can to improve our diet and lifestyle and give ourselves an opportunity to live a long and healthy life so we can be of the greatest benefit. The importance of breathing correctly is now coming to the forefront in the world of healthcare, longevity, and wellness. Research is now showing that breathing correctly might be even more important than what we eat. Studies on breathing show that the majority of people don't know how to breathe properly, and this is often the start of their health problems. We encourage you to explore the basic breathing techniques in chapter four to establish the foundation for the vase breath retention in the yoga of Niguma, but also to breathe more effectively throughout your day, and always through the nose. By doing so, you will not only become physically healthier, but you will be able to calm your emotions and find clarity of mind.

Lastly, make every effort to get enough sleep. Dream yoga and clear-light yoga practices are part of the six Dharmas of Niguma. Although we are not teaching those here, you can begin to prepare for these practices by improving your sleep hygiene. There are many wonderful resources on improving sleep and getting deep rest and dream time at night, including *Why We Sleep: Unlocking the Power of Sleep and Dreams* by Matthew Walker and *This Is Why You Dream: What Your Sleeping Brain Reveals About Your Waking Life* by Rahul Jandial.

PRACTICE MATERIALS

Niguma yoga is best practiced on a thick, padded, square cushion called a zabuton, which is approximately three feet wide on each side. We find that the most comfortable mat is a 100 cm by 100 cm six-layered version, which provides extra padding. If you don't have a zabuton, you can also use a bouldering crash pad or dense wool blankets covered by a hatha yoga sticky mat. A round zafu cushion is not necessary for this practice. To practice the preparatory stretches from hatha yoga that are included in this book and in our online resources, you'll need a standard hatha yoga sticky mat, a yoga block, and a yoga strap or belt.

Part 3
The Yoga of Niguma

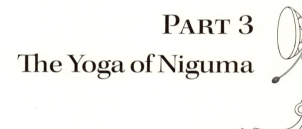

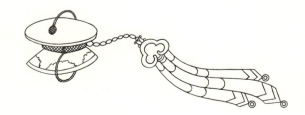

4

Building Your Niguma Yoga Practice

THE IMPORTANCE OF THE BREATH AND CONSISTENT PRACTICE

The yoga of Niguma is primarily a breathing practice for transformation. By focusing on the breath again and again as you inhale, exhale, and keep the air retained, heat and bliss are generated. And after a while, the mind becomes less fixated on sense objects, emotions, and physical sensations, and one enters the middle state of mind, which is a state of inner peace and equanimity.

If you can gently, gently, gently practice over time at staying present with the breath and retaining the breath, you will begin to overcome sensorial triggers, and then at the emotional level there will be fewer projections and negative reactions, such as anger and jealousy. There will be more wisdom, clarity, tolerance, and dissolution of negative patterns. As you progress in practice, negative reactions become less and less. But this takes time. In the beginning, working at dissolving layers of ego is like parenting a child. You must keep pointing out and explaining why they shouldn't behave this way. But with strong yoga and breathing awareness, you need less explanation and there is more instant recognition of the emotional trigger, and you can dissolve it in the moment.

If you practice yoga and breathing well and cultivate a resilient, clear, and truly compassionate mind, then you can truly be skillful when faced with realities of life and its ups and downs.

Be patient, consistently practice, and you will develop skills over time to find great happiness and freedom.

The practices described below will help you develop the foundational postures and breathing that are core to Niguma yoga, including how to build the vase breath and hatha yoga breathing practices that can provide additional support.

Foundational Posture and Breathing

The posture in which we begin and end all exercises is the vajra posture, also called full lotus or *padmasana*. Until the hips open, you can alternatively sit in a loose, cross-legged position on the floor or with ankles crossed sitting on the edge of a chair with your spine straight.* Once the hips open, you can sit in the traditional vajra posture with legs crossed on a zabuton cushion on the ground.

Extend your arms so they are straight and place your hands on your knees. The back should be straight, but also relaxed. The mind begins to settle into meditative awareness as you begin to notice your breath. Spend a few minutes relaxing into awareness. Allow any distracted thoughts and projections to dissolve away. Tell yourself, "Everything is impermanent, and therefore everything is perfect." Invite desire, fear, anger, or anything else that is clouding your mind to begin to float away into a clear sky of spacious awareness.

Breathe in and out through the nose throughout your practice.

In between each pose that follows, come back into this foundational meditative posture and take at least three breaths. Focus on the gap, or pause, at the end of each exhale to further relax the body and mind.

---

* Please see the appendix for instructions on getting into lotus/vajra posture and a complete series of hip opening postures to support building it.

Vajra Fists

When breathing in, the hands form a "vajra fist." Place the tip of each thumb at the base of the ring finger and close the hands into a fist. This hand position calms and focuses the mind and is said to reduce ignorance. It also protects and concentrates our vital energy inside the body and keeps negative energy from entering.

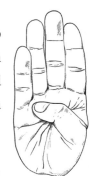

As the mind stills, we have a greater ability to hold a longer vase breath, which brings more clarity and transformational wisdom energy. While breathing out, open the hands in a relaxed way. The hands follow the flow of the breath.

Arrow Breathing and Vase Breath

Before starting an exercise, release stale air and energy from the body by performing an arrow breath and then fill and hold a vase breath throughout the duration of the posture.

Arrow Breath in Preparation for Vase Breath Before a Pose

In preparation for each exercise, take three breaths through the nose, opening and closing the hands with each breath. On the third exhale, perform a strong arrow breath. The arrow breath starts with a smooth exhale out the nose, like an arrow gliding through the air, then at the last moment, the exhalation comes out forcefully and audibly, like an arrow hitting its target. This forced exhale through the nose removes dead air, toxins, and tension, and creates an engagement and muscular toning of the pubococcygeus muscles at the center of the pelvic floor and the transversus abdominis in the lower abdominal region. This muscular toning is important for creating the fuller diaphragmatic vase breath that will soon follow. It also begins to pull up the lower wind energy toward the naval, which is important for cultivating heat and creating an experience of bliss. At the bottom of the arrow breath, open your hands so the fingers are outstretched. This is followed by a vase breath.

Vase Breathing

Vase breathing (Skt. *kumbhaka*; Tib. བུམ་པ་ཅན་, *bumpachen*) is a breathing technique that fills the pot of the belly, like filling a water vase from the base up to the narrow open top. The breath is most fully concentrated in the widest part of the container in the belly and it is held there to increase and stabilize one's vital energies or inner subtle winds (Skt. *vayu*; Tib. རླུང་, *lung*).

The exercises of Niguma yoga are accompanied by a vase breath to purify and direct the vital wind energies from the side channels of the energetic subtle body to the central channel, which balances the body/mind complex and creates wisdom, clarity, and bliss.

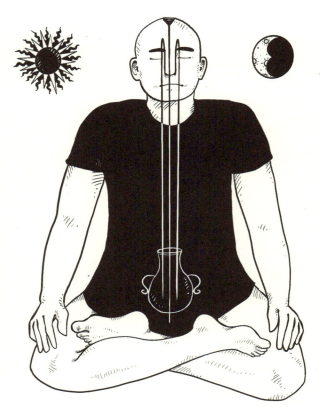

There are three main channels:

Central channel (Skt. *avadhuti*; Tib. དབུ་མ་, *uma*): Running from crown to base and parallel to the spine.

Solar channel (Skt. *rasana*; Tib. རོ་མ་, *roma*): To the right of the central channel.

Lunar channel left (Skt. *lalana*; Tib. རྐྱང་མ་, *kyangma*): To the left of the central channel.

There are five main winds:

Prana (Tib. སྲོག་གི་རླུང་, *rog gi lung*): The life-sustaining wind energy that is concentrated in the heart and lives at the center of the body; it governs mind and body and regulates the respiratory and cardiovascular systems. It is connected to the air element.

Samana (Tib. མེ་མཉམ་གྱི་རླུང་, *me nyam gi lung*): The wind energy connected to the fire element that ignites as the other winds are balanced and the opposing wind energies, prana and apana, are brought together at the navel. Samana vayu governs digestion and assimilation, and when it is fully active it creates bliss. Serotonin is produced in this area of the stomach and intestines, the home of samana vayu.

Udana (Tib. གྱེན་རྒྱུ་, *gyen gyu lung*): The ascending wind energy connected to the space element that lives in the throat and governs speech, eating, and drinking; it moves up and out.

Vyana (Tib. ཁྱབ་བྱེད་ཀྱི་རླུང་, *khyabje kyi lung*): The wind energy that controls all motor functions of the body. It starts in the heart, expands out to the limbs, and pervades the entire body. Its flow is governed by the water element.

Apana (Tib. ཐུར་སེལ་, *thur sel*): The descending wind associated with the earth element. Apana resides below the navel, primarily at the pelvic floor, and governs the process of elimination in the body.

Each Niguma yoga sequence works on purifying, increasing, and directing these vital subtle body energy winds. For each sequence in this book, we have highlighted some of the key subtle body effects to help you engage with them in your practice and recognize them when their transformative effect is encountered through ongoing practice.

Vase Breathing Technique

At the end of the arrow breath, take a very quick half-second long yet fully diaphragmatic in-breath to fill your belly and torso with air. The quick nature of this breath keeps you from taking the breath too high into the upper chest. The breath should stop about the level of the heart. The belly and torso are expanded in all directions, up to the top of the diaphragm. Once established, slightly pull up the pelvic floor muscles to create a lift below the vase and then press down from the top of the diaphragm or heart toward the navel to create a more expansive vase. It can help to swallow a little when you are first learning to press down from above. This quick breath, and the action of drawing up and pushing down, concentrates the wind energies into the pot of the belly around the level of our navel, where it should be held. Over time, it will become more refined and easier to hold.

Taking the breath up too high can create dizziness and too much wind energy. When pulling up the pelvic floor, try not to contract the belly muscles near the navel. The lowest belly muscles, four finger-widths below the navel, can simultaneously contract with the perineum muscles, but nothing higher.

As you are performing an exercise, if the vase breath begins to lessen, you can top it off with another quick puff of breath to return the fullness to your vase.

Over time with practice, the vase breath retention will be more comfortable to hold for longer periods. One should be relaxed, so don't force yourself to hold the breath longer than you're ready for.

Arrow Breath upon Completion of a Pose

Upon completing a pose, one returns to a crossed-legged position with hands on the knees and exhales forcefully with a quick arrow breath. This happens with the breath and hands in sync with one another. As the breath shoots out, the vajra fists land on the knees. As the arrow breath lands, the fingers fully extend out. The thumbs remain at the base of each ring finger. Hold the exhalation out as comfortably and long as possible to calm the nervous system. When the inhalation arises, close the vajra fists. When exhaling, open the palms and fingers. Focus on the pauses between each breath and the mind's luminosity and clarity.

Contraindications for Breath Retention
Pregnancy (pregnant women should only do very short breath retentions, if at all); high blood pressure that is not controlled; heart disease; and lung disease.

SIMPLE BREATHING PRACTICES THAT PROMOTE RELAXATION AND PREPARE FOR THE VASE BREATH

As you begin your journey with the yoga of Niguma, it is important to understand how to breathe correctly and access the muscles we use to create a full vase breath.

Aligned breathing is the most powerful medicine for longevity and restores our physical health and happiness, and can elevate us to higher levels of consciousness. Practice the foundational breathing techniques below to have a deeper understanding of how to breathe, relax, and build your capacity to perform a vase breath.

Yogic Breathing

Prana is the creative life force within us and the fluid energy that is in our breath and sustains all of our bodily systems. It is also intimately connected to the mind, the two informing each other. The highest state of an awakened mind is equated to the finest prana. The mind discovers its natural state of bliss and luminosity as the breath is refined and prana is freed to flow expansively within the body. Our yoga practice helps to liberate and direct prana by opening the physical and subtle body channels and increasing our awareness. As this happens, mental obscurations are also cleared. One of the first steps toward liberating our life force and improving our health is to simply observe our body breathing and learn how to make full use of the natural diaphragmatic breathing process.

Many of us don't know how to breathe effectively and therefore can't engage with this life force fully. For beginners of Niguma yoga and yoga practitioners in general, I highly recommend you spend time exploring the symphony of muscles in your body that work together to take a full diaphragmatic breath. Each Niguma yoga posture utilizes a vase breath, and for it to be the support and powerful tool needed to safely and correctly perform each pose, you must be able to access all the working parts of your remarkable breathing apparatus.

Intermediate students can utilize this practice to gain deeper insight and control of your subtle body channels and wind energies. Below are some preparatory exercises that will support your overall health and prepare you for taking the vase breath used in Niguma yoga.

The Diaphragm

It is important to also understand how our diaphragm muscle moves.

During an inhalation, our dome-shaped diaphragm muscle contracts, flattens, and moves inferiorly, causing our abdominal muscles to move downward toward the pelvis. As a result, the belly should expand out and the side body should widen out, increasing the diameter of the thorax as your ribs take an excursion laterally. When you watch a child breathing naturally, you will see the wave-like movement of the breath expanding their belly like a balloon. Adults most often lose this natural belly movement from chronic tension and holding in their belly region, whether from stress, standing for long periods, emotional trauma, or otherwise. We must learn to free the belly during the vase breath and only draw up the muscles of the pelvic floor and the lower fibers of our transversus abdominis muscles, which are nearer the pubic bone and a few inches up. The navel area should not be held in.

The practices that follow enhance and give us insight into the practice of taking a deep diaphragmatic breath.

Constructive Rest Pose

The constructive rest pose is powerful for relaxation and cultivating intimacy with the symphony of muscles in your body that work together to take a full diaphragmatic breath, which is essential for being able to do the vase breath in Niguma yoga.

This practice can also help us understand how to activate the muscles used in what hatha yoga calls uddiyana bandha and mula bandha. *Bandha* is Sanskrit for binding, catching, or drawing up into one's awareness. Mula bandha involves the contraction of the perineal muscles and the drawing of one's attention to the perineum's center point, just in front of the anus and behind the genitals. It is essentially a meditative awakening at what feels to be the root of the body (*mula*) done in conjunction with the breath. Uddiyana bandha is a complementary contraction to mula bandha that draws up the perineum and draws back the lower belly, just above the pubic bone. It lifts the abdominal organs up off the pelvic floor and provides stability to the spine and abdomen so that a full inhalation can occur. The hatha yoga bandhas are similarly applied in Niguma yoga after taking a vase breath by drawing up the perineum and lifting the area four finger-widths below and behind the navel. This movement is often incorrectly performed by pulling in the navel area or pelvic floor too strongly, which compromises the fullness of the vase breath. Mula bandha is more closely connected with letting go and staying present for the natural contraction that occurs at the bottom of the exhalation. It is a state of surrender, renunciation, connection to emptiness, and dissolving, rather than something you forcefully apply. If you just follow the breath to completion, the pelvic floor and lower belly will automatically contract. As you practice constructive rest pose, stay present for these natural contractions that occur as you observe the ends of the breath.

Moving into the Pose

1. Lie down on your back with your legs bent to ninety degrees and your arms by your side. You can march the legs up and down a few times until the feet and knees land on the ground in a position just right for you. The lower back should have a natural, soft curve; don't try to make it flat.

2. Place your hands on your belly to begin to feel the rise and fall of your natural breath. Allow your belly to simply expand as you inhale and fall back toward the earth as you exhale. Stay present for the complete length of your inhalation. Stay present for the full extension of your exhalation. Notice the tone of the muscles of the lower belly and base of your spine as you complete each breath cycle.

3. Stay for five to ten minutes and remain completely absorbed in your breathing process and the sensations that arise with the breath movement. As you continue to be present for each breath, become familiar with the luminosity of mind and relaxation response that accompanies this witnessing. Mind and breath go together. When we find space and a soft fluidity in our breathing, our mind aligns and becomes spacious awareness.

Variations

If you are carrying stress or have back tightness or pain, focus on letting your belly expand on each inhalation and your lower back releasing toward the ground on each exhalation. Your lower back will softly begin to move toward the ground as you relax. Let this happen naturally with the breath without trying to press the back down. Rather just witness how the breath's natural wave patterns will create the shift.

Notice the sensations in the body as your breath flows in and reaches the upper crest of the wave. Notice the gaps between each breath and the gaps in thought, just spacious presence that happens in the space between each breath. Just by tuning in, we begin to connect the upper and lower wind energies as relational—not truly in opposition, but rising out of each other. We can experience a feeling of emptiness at the bottom of the exhalation and boundlessness at the top of the inhalation. These are in fact two ends of the same stick, and although they produce different sensations and appear uniquely, they are eventually seen as part of an interconnected whole.

Subtle Body Highlights

Constructive rest pose is a basic yet powerful mindfulness practice, an active form of shamatha, or calm-abiding meditation, that will help to cultivate the wisdom of emptiness and even prepare us for perfection stage practice in Vajrayana, which includes drop yoga and subtle body yoga, the yoga practices of blissful merging and melting the subtle essence within the upper and lower drops throughout the chakras and together at the heart.

Once you become more familiar with the subtle energy in the body via concentrated awareness, you will also understand why Niguma constructed her series the way she did. Getting up from the ground, you feel the lower winds being pulled up into the upper, and sitting back down, you might notice the upper being poured into the lower. Each sequence is working on a different energy channel and wind energy. And the elegant and sophisticated way Niguma balances and transforms the body is awe inspiring.

Yogic traditions say the body and mind are inseparable; the chitta (mind) is always together with prana (energy/winds). Where one goes, the other follows, or rather travels alongside. Know that as you focus your awareness on your belly breathing, energy will begin to flow to that focal point.

The belly is the home of samana vayu, a wind energy in your body that awakens as we unite opposing patterns and cultivate equanimity. An experienced yogi learns to take the wind energy prana vayu, which lives in the heart and normally moves up and out in the direction of the crown of the head, and reverse its natural flow, taking it down to the navel. Likewise, the experienced yogi takes the lower wind, apana vayu, which normally resides in the pelvic floor and moves down and out with the exhale, and redirects this flow to the navel. Bringing together the upper and lower winds (prana and apana) and wakening samana vayu are key in building the tummo fire called chandali, *which in turn is key in activating the body's enlightening process.*

Subtle body yoga requires an intimacy with the natural flow of the wind energies in your body. Practice being keenly attentive to your breath movement and the natural gaps between each breath, and the ability to redirect the flow will naturally arise.

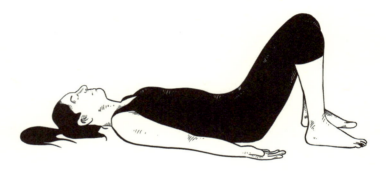

Seated Yoga Breathing for Diaphragmatic Awareness

Take a comfortable cross-legged seat on the ground or edge of a chair. Use elevation as needed to allow your pelvis to be neutral and your spine to lengthen. Align your pelvic floor with your palate and the center of your head. Keeping a straight spine, practice deep breaths, allowing your belly to expand to the sides and fill the belly like a balloon. Create as much space as you can without creating tension from your efforts. Fill from the top of the belly down to the pelvic floor and let your lower side ribs move out while you expand your abdomen. After several rounds of full breath, imagine that you are equally filling a vase with fluid from the base up. Then keenly become aware of the ends of the breath. You might notice the pelvic floor relax down at the top of your inhalation and contract in and up at the bottom of your exhalation. Stay present with the ends of the breath and the sensations that arise in these gaps between inhaling and exhaling. Perform three, seven, fourteen, or twenty-one rounds.

Viloma Pranayama

I (Michele) chose to include this wonderful pranayama technique because of the way that Kalu Rinpoche teaches filling the vase breath and topping off the vase breath. He stresses to do a very fast fill for two seconds or so into the belly and chest, but not too high. Taking it too high can cause dizziness. I am so grateful for this instruction, as I often became dizzy when instructed by other teachers due to filling so high. Then, as the breath starts to seep out while Rinpoche is performing a sequence, he will take a quick sip of breath to keep the fullness, but again, not too high. By practicing viloma pranayama, we can get a sense of what he is doing as we too practice filling, stopping, and then filling some more. *Viloma* means cutting or snipping hair in Sanskrit. Here, you cut the torso into three or four parts, sometimes more, and breathe in, pause, breathe in a little more, pause, and then a little more, and so on. You can practice it as you move the inhalation up, and it can be also practiced as you are exhaling down.

Technique

Viloma pranayama can be done sitting or lying down in constructive rest pose, or lying down on the ground supine with legs outstretched and with a bolster supporting the length of the back and head in what is called savasana 2 (corpse pose with bolster) position. I like to divide the torso into three parts, but you can do more.

1. Breathe into the lower belly, then stop. Hold for a few seconds.
2. Add a little more and breathe into the upper belly, then stop. Hold for a few seconds.
3. Add a little more and breathe into the chest, then stop. Hold for a few seconds, and then breathe all the way out.

Pranayama Utilizing 1:2 Ratio

Kalu Rinpoche stresses that if after finishing a Niguma yoga sequence we find our breathing pace increased and adrenaline flowing as a residue of the sequence, we should focus on softly lengthening our exhalation as well as the pause after the exhalation. When I was first learning the Niguma yoga postures, especially the first third of the poses, my heart rate would increase significantly and I would want to reach for an inhalation, sometimes even gasp for a breath. But upon Rinpoche's guidance to hold out the exhalation, I quickly learned the wisdom behind his instruction. It is indeed the fastest way to return to a state of equilibrium and calm the bodily processes.

To support our ability to extend the exhalation, I suggest we train with a technique I learned from the wonderful Kaivalyadhama lineage of pranayama masters who have done leading research on the benefits of pranayama and cultivating a 1:2 ratio of inhalation to exhalation when practicing pranayama.

An example of 1:2 ratio would be to inhale for five counts and exhale for ten. If that is too difficult, reduce to a four-count inhalation and eight-count exhalation, or less. This can be done when practicing alternating nostril breathing (nadis shodhana), other pranayama exercises, or just simply while doing deep diaphragmatic breathing. Strengthening the capacity to extend the exhalation will help you to be more grounded as well.

Technique

1. Sit with your spine straight in meditation posture and place the tip of your tongue at the root of your upper front teeth. Draw up the perineum gently and take the gaze down the nose softly. Relax your chin toward your heart and lift your heart toward your chin.

2. Inhale and take a vase breath for four or five counts. Exhale for eight or ten counts.

3. Pay particular attention to the natural gap at the bottom of your exhalation

and the natural gap at the top of your inhalation. Increase the length of the breath and the ratio as you become more adept at breathing out in a relaxed way.

Part III
The Yoga of Niguma

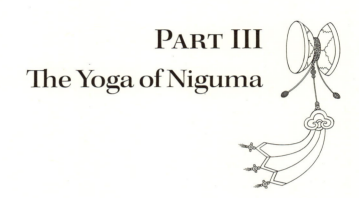

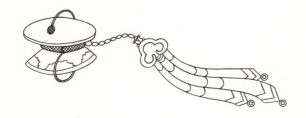

5

The Yoga of Niguma Sequences: Illustrations and Instructions

NIGUMA YOGA SEQUENCE 1

Freeing the Knots in the Channels

Moving in the Sequence

1. Sit in the vajra posture, or establish a simple cross-legged seat on a flat cushion or at the edge of a chair.
2. Prepare with the three breaths, as explained above in "Foundational Vajra Posture and Breathing" (see page 32). Finish with an arrow breath.
3. Establish your vase breath and hold throughout the duration of this posture.
4. Take your vajra fists from their position on the knees and slide them along the sides of your crossed legs smoothly up to land at the top of your thighs. Press the vajra fist palm down into the center of your thigh, just in front of your groin. Your knuckles face each other toward the center of your body's midline.
5. Push the vajra fists down into your thighs and straighten your arms. The upper arms should be squeezing in so they are as straight as possible.
6. Look straight ahead and try not to move the head, just the torso.

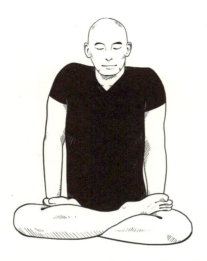 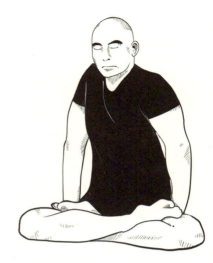

7. Starting with the right side, throw the right side of the torso toward the left knee forcefully seven times. Keep your shoulders back and your chest lifted, so the movement remains a twisting action for the torso, rather than a shoulder movement. If necessary, you can top off your breath now, before switching sides, to create the full vase.
8. Repeat the movement from the left side. The torso twists to the right and springs back into place seven times.
9. After the torso twists to each side, slide your vajra fists along the outside of the thighs so they return to the tops of the knees. Once they land, release the breath via an arrow breath, extend the fingers, and calmly breathe.

Precautions and Contraindications
Pregnancy, disc injuries, sacroiliac joint injuries, and carpal tunnel syndrome.

Preparatory Postures
Spinal twists from hatha yoga, hip openers, and wrist exercises for strength and mobility.

Subtle Body Highlights
This exercise purifies the right and left channels and pours opposing pattern energy from the sun and moon channels, masculine and feminine, together to create equilibrium and bliss.

NIGUMA YOGA SEQUENCE 1 SUPPORTING PRACTICES

Niguma yoga sequence 1 powerfully twists each side of the body for spinal mobility and clears the energetic subtle body side channels, untying knots within them. To prepare for this rapid and strong bodily movement, we can regularly practice holding gentle twists to increase the range of motion of the spine and stretch the muscles of the back, ribs, and shoulders progressively.

Practice the gentle basic seated twists below to prepare the spine with focused inhalations and exhalations. Hold the twist for twenty seconds to each side to allow the muscles to open. It is a very simple yet powerful technique to assist the spine and abdominal organs to find health and mobility.

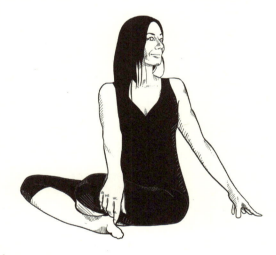

Seated Twist 1

Moving into the Pose
1. Establish a cross-legged seat or sit at the edge of a chair.
2. Place the left hand to the side of the left hip or hold the edge of the chair. Root down through the sitting bones and push through the hand to lengthen the spine.
3. Inhale and further lengthen the spine up from the pelvis while establishing a subtle lift at the pelvic floor and lower belly.

4. Exhale and twist your upper belly and torso to the left, taking your right hand to the outside of your left knee.

5. Inhale again to lengthen the spine and exhale to twist deeper. As the upper torso and head follow the direction of the twist, allow the lower belly to counter twist slightly in the opposite direction, which will provide core support. The right hand's fingers spread and root into the floor or your support behind you, creating a tent shape with the hand to guide the lift of the spine.

6. Softly gaze at a single point with wide peripheral vision and allow the twist to deepen with each breath. Stay at least five breaths.

When we twist, we should lift the perineum and contract the pit of the abdomen to support the spine and sacrum. For a classic twist with mindful breathing, take a deep inhalation and then exhale fully to tone the muscles at the base of the spine and pelvic floor. Keep the tone, then inhale to lengthen the spine, and then exhale to move into the twist. Each exhalation can deepen the twist. Each inhalation can provide more length to the spine and space between the vertebrae. For these preparatory twists, we can allow the breath's intelligent wave pattern to guide us in the pose and move us deeper when the spine is ready. Allow your head to follow the spine's movement rather than letting the head lead. Once in the full twist, soften your gaze to a single point and allow the peripheral vision to widen. Lift the palate from the tongue and create a feeling in the mouth that resembles saying "ahh," or feeling awe.

Seated Twist 2: Ardha Matsyendrasana (Half Lord of the Fishes)

This twist increases spinal, hip, shoulder, and neck mobility while improving digestion and circulation to the abdominal region and spinal discs. This twist automatically brings in core activation to protect the lower back, and slight flexion to protect the sacroiliac joint that connects the pelvis and spine. Regular practice will not only bring ease to your Niguma yoga twists, it will also help you open up the legs and hips to improve your sitting posture.

Moving into the Pose

1. Establish a cross-legged seat and cross your right knee over your left to place your right foot standing on the ground next to your left knee. If this is not accessible, perform the posture with a straight left leg.
2. Tent the fingers of your right hand to the ground just behind your right hip. Root down through the hand to lift your spine.
3. Take a big inhalation and extend your left arm up into the air to elongate the entire side body and spine, lifting the pit of the abdomen.
4. Exhale and take the arm across the right leg to hook the left elbow to the outside of the right leg.
5. Press into the leg with your arm to leverage the twist. Continue to root down to the earth with the feet, pelvis, and hand to lengthen your spine. The belly moves into the twist first, and then the rest of the torso with the head slowly follows the rest of the spine.
6. Gaze off into space softly with wide peripheral vision and breathe deeply and completely for at least five breaths.

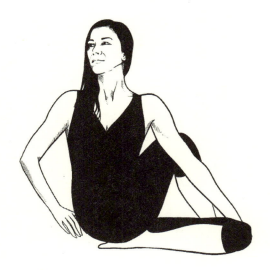

NIGUMA YOGA SEQUENCE 2
Straightening the Channels

The second Niguma yoga sequence is the first of many that takes us from the vajra posture, the cross-legged seat, to standing and then back to a seat again. After completing a cycle of arrow breathing and establishing a vase breath, one performs a *shik*, also called "breaking the posture."

Shik (Breaking the Posture)

To release the vajra posture, before standing or moving into a pose that requires free legs, we break the posture. This is a graceful movement of the arms that coordinates the arms lifting, crossing, and landing on the knees with an unwinding of the vajra legs.

Moving in the Sequence

1. Keeping the thumbs at the base of the ring finger, lift the arms up in front of the chest with the right arm further away from your torso.
2. Cross the right arm in front of the left, pull the hands through the space between the arms, and briskly land the outstretched arms and the vajra fists on each knee. At the same time, the legs unwind from the vajra posture.
3. As the knees and feet touch the ground, the fists land on the knees.

Bep (Controlled Fall or Mindful Transition to a Seat)

A careful transition from standing postures back to a vajra seat is done in many of the Niguma sequences. The traditional way to do this transition is via a vajra drop, or controlled fall, called a *bep*. One must learn how to do a bep correctly directly in person from an expert teacher to receive personal guidance in the technique. Please do not try a bep without in-person instruction. One must learn how to strike the ground correctly, hitting the thighs and buttocks evenly and always with the breath retained. The vase breath retention cushions the spine in the fall and is essential to prevent injury. Until you have proper instruction, train by keeping the vase breath held as you simply cross your feet, bend your knees, and slowly sit down. The bep has the purpose of moving the subtle body energetic winds through the channels and directing them into the central channel to promote higher states of awareness, clarity, and bliss.

Moving in the Sequence

1. Keeping the vase breath, break the posture, stand up, and place your vajra fists on your front hip bones.
2. Move your hips and belly in circles with a hula-hoop action to the right three times and to the left three times.
3. Extend your arms along your sides.
4. Lift your heels up and rock to the ball mounds of your feet and then drop the heels back down for a heel drop.
5. Carefully cross your feet and lower yourself to a seat and then stand up again while retaining the breath. If you have been trained by a master in the bep drop technique, perform a bep to your vajra seat and then stand up again. This will be done seven times.
6. Each time you stand, do a quick heel drop and then transition back to the ground.

THE YOGA OF NIGUMA SEQUENCES: ILLUSTRATIONS AND INSTRUCTIONS 57

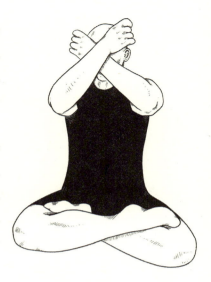

7. As you take each seat, cross your arms just like you do with the shik, right outside the left, and pull them through. This graceful movement of the arms is coordinated so one strikes the ground with the legs while simultaneously landing the vajra fists on the knees.
8. Most importantly, the vase breath must be retained the entire time. If you lose the vase breath, stop what you are doing and establish it once more. The vase breath protects the spine and pelvis and all the internal organs. It also cushions the spinal discs.
9. At the end of the seven beps, finish in a relaxed cross-legged posture and release the vase breath with an arrow breath.
10. Go into a meditative mode and focus on extending the pause after each exhalation to calm the nervous system and heart rate, and slow your breathing. With each exhalation, open your hands and extend your fingers. With each inhalation, close your hands in a vajra fist.

Precautions and Contraindications
Present knee injuries or knee pain, disc injuries, and severe osteoarthritis in the hip joints.

Preparations
Standing poses to build leg and knee strength from hatha yoga and hip opening poses; see the appendix.

Subtle Body Highlights
This exercise builds and raises the chandali (or inner fire) at the base of the body. Chandali is also Sanskrit for "fierce woman." It increases adrenaline and the sun energy, helping to move the winds up into the central channel (Skt. sushumna) to increase bliss.

NIGUMA YOGA SEQUENCE 2 SUPPORTING PRACTICES

An important sign of health and longevity is the ability to stand up from the ground without using your hands. Called the "floor predictor," modern scientific research has shown that this musculoskeletal fitness indicator is accurate at determining all-cause mortality (general causes of death in a population). This Niguma sequence builds our capacity to stand from the ground by building our glutes and leg muscles and challenges us to strengthen our cardiovascular system even more due to the addition of the vase breath. Scientific studies on heart disease have also shown a correlation between weakness in the thigh muscles and weakness in the heart.

Niguma yoga sequence 2 and the other sequences that require rising from the ground are the most challenging yet rewarding sequences. They increase adrenaline, and with regular practice, the yogi quickly notices improvement in their cardiovascular system and leg strength.

If you are not able to stand up with ease, you can do this exercise from the seat of a chair. But it is also recommended you build leg, glute, and knee strength and stability by working on squats, lunges, resistance training, and the hatha yoga postures that strengthen the thighs. Warrior 2 (virabhadrasana 2), the side angle pose (parsvakonasana), chair pose (utkatasana), and variations of these are very helpful in building thigh strength. They also safely open the groin and hips while increasing the external rotation and mobility in the hips that is required for the vajra posture. These lunges strengthen the knees as we work toward a ninety-degree bend accompanied by good knee to foot alignment. Students with knee issues can have difficulty standing from the ground with crossed legs, and it might increase their pain. The hatha yoga standing poses can support rehabilitation from knee injuries and increase mobility to make this practice possible.

THE YOGA OF NIGUMA SEQUENCES: ILLUSTRATIONS AND INSTRUCTIONS   59

Recommended Standing Postures:

Virabhadrasana 2: Warrior 2
Parsvakonasana: Side angle
Trikonasana: Triangle pose
Ardha chandrasana: Half-moon pose
Utkatasana: Chair pose
Utkata konasana: Goddess pose

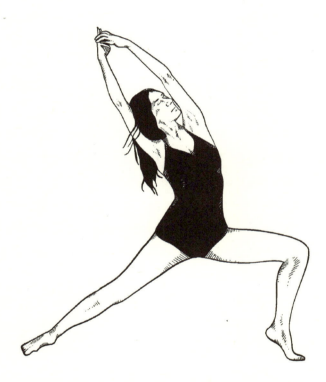

*Practice lifting your heels in controlled warrior poses to build arch and knee strength and draw up the lower wind or apana vital wind energy. This will help you find more height when performing the heel lifts and drops that are found in many of the Niguma yoga sequences.

Virabhadrasana 2 (Warrior 2)

Moving into the Pose

1. Step your feet out wide apart, about the distance of one of your legs plus a half leg more. In hatha yoga terminology this is called a leg and a half leg stance. Turn your right foot out ninety degrees, parallel with the long edge of your mat, and turn the left foot in fifteen degrees. Align the second toe mound and the center of the right heel with the front of the left heel. From deep within the right hip socket, rotate the right leg externally so the knee aligns with the second toe. Rotate the femur from the hip, not the ankle.

2. Take an inhalation and draw the prana vital wind energy into the body, pull up the sheaths of the legs, lift the pit of the abdomen, and lift the pelvis up off the femurs. Drop and spread the shoulder blades.

3. Exhale as you bend the right knee to ninety degrees, tracking it straight in alignment with the right second toe mound. The thighbone and shinbone should form a right angle, with the shinbone perpendicular to the floor. The left heel presses strongly into the ground and the back leg—that is, the left leg—is straight as the left quadricep presses back. Lift the front hip off of the femur. Ground down equally into the four corners of your feet, lift the arches and anklebones, and spread your toes.

4. Reach back with the left arm, resisting the collapse of the spine to the right.

5. Lift the pit of the abdomen, drop the shoulders, spread the upper back, and actively spread the arms. Turn your head and look at the second finger of your right hand.

6. Stay in the pose for five to ten breaths, breathing smoothly with a soft mouth and eyes.

7. Inhale and come out of the pose.

Prop Work

- *If you have balance issues or need extra support while training in this pose, you can place the front thigh over the seat of a chair.*

- *To assist staying centered and build shoulder alignment and strength, you can press your back hand into a wall.*
- *If there is pain in your back leg's foot due to a tight Achilles tendon or calf, you can place your back foot's heel at the wall or place a quarter round or pad under the back heel to reduce any discomfort.*

Benefits

This pose has several benefits, including opening the hips; grounding the body and mind energetically by purifying the lower wind energy of apana, which is connected to the earth element; building confidence; and strengthening the legs, abdomen, lower back, and heart.

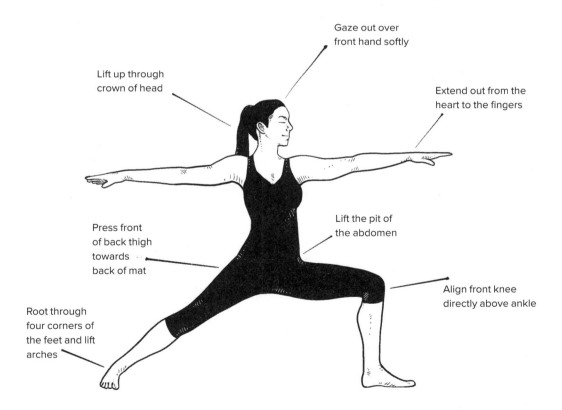

NIGUMA YOGA SEQUENCE 3

Gathering into the Uma

~~~~~~

Moving in the Sequence

1. Sit in the vajra posture, perform a cycle of arrow breathing, and establish a vase breath.
2. Break the posture with the shik.
3. Stand up quickly, with arms by your side and each hand in a vajra fist.
4. Do two quick heel drops and then one small jump into the air, landing down on both feet.
5. Repeat this pattern seven times.
6. Directly after landing the seventh lift, confirm the vase breath is established soundly. Then cross the arms and do a standing bep or carefully sit back down on the ground.
7. The vajra fists land on the knees at the moment your legs simultaneously sit on the ground.
8. Upon landing, release the vase breath with an arrow breath exhalation.
9. Relax and calm the body and breath by focusing on extending the exhalation.

Precautions and Contraindications

Severe bunions that limit heel raises, present knee injuries or knee pain, disc injuries, and severe osteoarthritis in hip joints.

Preparations

Standing poses to build leg and knee strength from hatha yoga and hip opening; see the appendix.

Subtle Body Highlights

The channels (Skt. nadi; Tib. ᚊ, tsa) are rivers or paths in the body for the flow of vital energy. Both hatha yoga and Vajrayana yoga systems, like that of Niguma, say that there are 7,200 channels in the body, along with a central channel.

A primary goal of yoga is the gathering and moving of the wind energies from the outer channels into the central channel. Heel lifts and drops help to lift the arches of the feet, which in turn activates the muscles of the legs and pelvic floor. The pelvic floor is home to the downward wind energy of apana, which governs elimination. As the heels drop in this pose, the energy that normally flows down will rebound up. Like bouncing a ball on the floor, our energy lifts up the central channel toward the crown of the head.

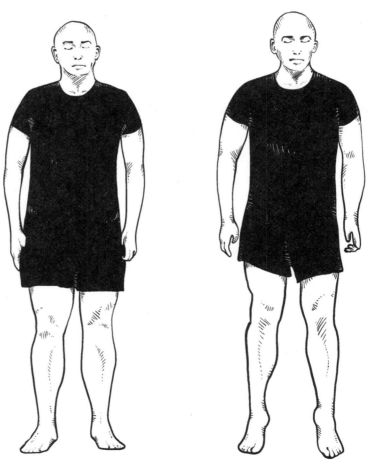

NIGUMA YOGA SEQUENCE 4
Spreading Out Through the Channels

Moving in the Sequence

1. Sit in the vajra posture, perform a cycle of arrow breathing, and establish a vase breath.
2. Open your palms and stretch out all your fingers while keeping the thumb at the base of the ring finger, then pat the head from the forehead up and over the crown to the back of the head and upper neck and then back to front again.
3. Make a vajra fist with the left hand, stretch your right arm parallel to the ground, and tap the arm with the left fist from the top of the arm down to the wrist and back up the arm.
4. Open the palm and rub the arm a few times, sliding back and forth.
5. Repeat on the other side.

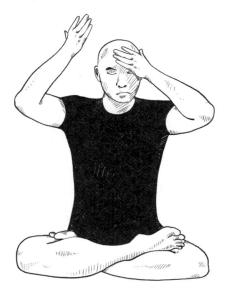
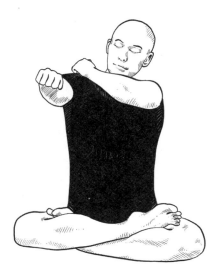

6. Break the posture, stretch out the right leg, and place the foot of the left bent leg on the inner part of the upper right thigh.
7. Massage the whole length of the leg with both open palms three times, from upper thigh to foot and back up. Each time you come up, lift your hands up high and then bow down with your whole torso until you slide from the upper thigh to the foot. This is a forward fold.
8. Repeat on the left leg.
9. When you finish the left side, quickly cross your legs and perform an arrow breath to release the vase.

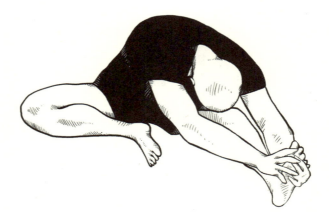

Precautions and Contraindications
Present knee injuries or knee pain, spinal disc injuries, or lumbar strain.

Preparations
Hip opening from hatha yoga and janu sirsasana. See the appendix for hip opening postures.

Subtle Body Highlights
This exercise supports the movement of the all-pervasive wind energy and moves blocked energy through the 7,200 channels. It purifies apana and spreads the drops (Skt. bindu; *Tib.* ཐིག་ལེ་, *thigle). A bindu is a seed of energy, a drop of enlightened*

mind, a point of rainbow light, and the essence of immutable great bliss. The bindus are also connected to the reproductive fluids of the father and mother: white in the head from the father, with the nature of luminosity, and red four fingers below and behind the navel from the mother, with the nature of radiance. A yogi will work with these seeds of energy to increase their potency, move them together, take them into the chakras, and spread their essence of boundless love, compassion, joy, equanimity, and wisdom throughout the body. This subtle body practice of blissfully melting and moving drops into the chakras and channels is called "drop yoga" and "subtle body yoga." Yoga keeps the bindu from drying up, and by circulating them throughout the body, the yogi's mind finds its natural state of well-being and happiness. When you are tapping and massaging the body in this sequence, feel that you are increasing and spreading their essence throughout your body.

NIGUMA SEQUENCE 4 SUPPORTING PRACTICE
Janu Sirsasana (Head-to-Knee Pose)

This Niguma yoga sequence uses janu sirsasana, or head-to-knee pose. On its own, this pose helps to open your hips and legs, massages the abdominal organs, and can build the vajra or lotus posture. It purifies the body as it focuses on the elimination pattern and downward winds of apana. It should be practiced until one has ease in folding over completely, with the knee resting firmly on the ground. If you have had knee surgery or injuries, the props suggested here can help support your recovery. Spending time in this pose daily will allow you to establish the external rotation needed in the lotus posture as well as bring flexibility to the legs and entire back body. Holding the pose for five to ten breaths or more calms the nervous system and improves digestion.

Moving into the Pose

1. Lean back with a posterior tilt to your pelvis and fold your right leg tightly closed, using both hands to create closure at the knee joint. Leaning back allows for the tightest closure of the knee joint, which is essential for the health of the knee.
2. If there is a gap at the knee crease, you can place a washcloth folded in a triangle shape tightly between the calf and knee.
3. Take the folded right leg out to the side and place the sole of the foot to the inseam of your straight left leg.
4. Shift the hips to square to even up the pelvis. To facilitate that, you can lift the straight leg's sit bone up and drag the leg back until your hips are square.
5. Twist your torso to the left and wrap the right waist toward the straight left leg. Twisting toward the straight leg is impor-

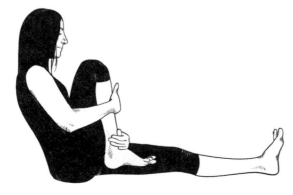

tant to open the hips as well as protect the sacroiliac joint, which connects the pelvis and spine, from strain.

6. If the bent knee is off the ground, you can place a firm cushion or block underneath the knee for support.

7. Engage the left quadriceps and press the left leg into the ground. Inhale and lift your arms up high into the air, lengthening the torso, side body, and spine as much as you can. Exhale and forward fold and catch the foot with your hands or a yoga strap or belt.

8. In the final form, hold the left foot with the palms facing out. The right hand will grab the left wrist, which allows you to leverage spinal extension. Stay for five breaths or more.

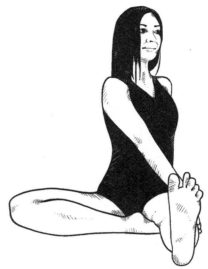

NIGUMA YOGA SEQUENCE 5
Standing and Spreading Through the Channels

Moving in the Sequence

1. Sit in the vajra posture, perform a cycle of arrow breathing, and establish a vase breath.
2. Break the posture and stand up quickly.
3. Keeping loose vajra fists, slide the hands up the side of the body, touching the side of the waist and chest. Then, from the level of the collarbone, slide the hands to the back of the neck and head, drawing a line up with fists together until they reach above the crown of the head.
4. Place the hands into a prayer position over the head and then bring them to hover just above the crown.

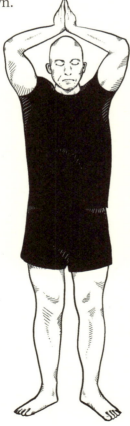

5. Jump into the air for seven quick hops. The hands stay in the prayer position.

6. Jump so that your feet leave the ground completely and land evenly back on the ground on the ball and heel equally.

7. Ensuring the vase breath is strongly established, release the posture with the classic hand break posture, then have a seat or perform a standing bep.

8. Finish the sequence in the seated vajra posture and complete the arrow breath. As the breath finishes, the hands land on the knees with fingers extending outward. The thumbs stay pressed to the base of the ring finger.

9. Focus on the bottom of the exhalation to calm the mind. Meditate on the mind's luminosity. The Buddha taught that the natural state of our mind is luminous and free from any defilements. When practicing yoga, especially after a sequence is finished or in the pause at the end of a breath when mental chatter has stilled, one can connect to the mind's natural state of pure luminous clarity.

Precautions and Contraindications
Present knee injuries or knee pain on standing, disc injuries, frozen shoulder, and rotator cuff tears.

Subtle Body Highlights
Hopping invites the apana vital wind energy to reverse its downward flow and move up toward the navel center. It also invites prana vital wind energy in turn to reverse and move down from its normal seat in the heart toward the navel. When these opposing winds meet at the navel, an alchemical process begins to form heat, which purifies obscurations in mind and body, raises creative energy, melts the subtle body drops (bindus), and promotes a return to our natural state of blissful luminous mind.

NIGUMA YOGA SEQUENCE 6
Moving the Limbs

Moving in the Sequence

1. Seated in the vajra posture, perform a cycle of arrow breathing and establish a vase breath.
2. Break the posture and stand up quickly.
3. Slide your right loose vajra fist up the center of the body to shoulder height, and with a smooth sweeping movement, outstretch the right arm slightly to the right to around 2 o'clock. The hand opens but the thumb stays to the base of the ring finger.
4. Simultaneously the right leg follows, lifting and extending to the same angle the arm is pointing.

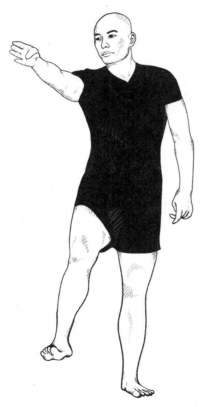

5. Pull the outstretched arm and leg vigorously into a flexed position, use the thumb-side of the right vajra fist to strike the right shoulder front, near the top of the arm bone and side of the chest on the pectoralis minor muscle. Then immediately spring it back to extend an outstretched arm and outstretched leg.

6. Pump and throw—that is, contract and extend—the arm and leg simultaneously three times.

7. Repeat the same on the left side.

8. Ensuring the vase breath is strongly established, release the posture with the classic hand break posture and either have a seat or perform a standing bep.

9. Finish the sequence in the seated vajra posture and complete the arrow breath. As the breath finishes, the hands land on the knees with fingers extending outward. The thumbs stay pressed to the base of the ring fingers.

10. Focus on the bottom of the exhalation to calm the mind and meditate on the mind's luminosity.

Note: If you wish, more than three strikes can be made. But remember to perform an equal number on each side.

Precautions and Contraindications

Balance issues due to traumatic brain injury or poor eyesight, vertigo, risk of falling due to pregnancy, and knee pain on compression.

Preparations

Balancing postures done at a wall and knee flexion poses from hatha yoga, such as child's pose, to build compression slowly.

Subtle Body Highlights

This sequence activates and purifies the tortoise channel, or kurma vayu, *in the rear channels of the body, which regulates extension and contraction of the limbs and is associated with the wind element.*

NIGUMA YOGA SEQUENCE 7
Pressing Down from the Upper Body

Moving in the Sequence

1. Seated in the vajra posture, perform one complete cycle of arrow breathing. Establish a vase breath and break the posture.
2. Stay seated with loose crossed legs. Slide the hands up the sides of the torso to chest level. Hook the thumbs inside the armpits and keep them there, and tightly interlock the fingers over the front of the chest.
3. Keeping your head in the forward position and back straight, put your elbows straight out to the sides. The arms will form a straight line that is level with the shoulders.
4. Throw the right shoulder forward using the upper torso as a fulcrum so the right elbow flings forward and the left elbow flings backward. Keeping your elbows and arms up at shoulder height, continue by throwing the left shoulder forward. Alternate right to left. By leading with the elbow tip, the other elbow will naturally turn and fulcrum backwards. Throw rigorously back and forth for seven rounds. You start and end with the right shoulder.
5. Finish by sitting in a relaxed cross-legged position with hands on knees. Complete the arrow breath while opening the hands.

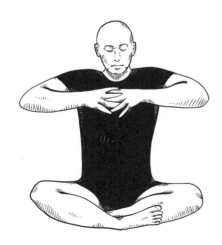
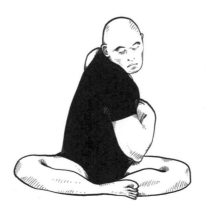
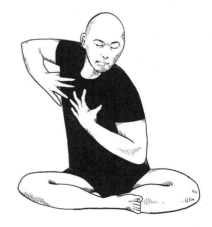

Precautions and Contraindications

Disc injuries, pregnancy, and sacroiliac joint instability.

Preparations

Hatha yoga twists, shoulder blade mobilization stretches, opposite elbow-to-knee standing oblique curls.

Subtle Body Highlights

This sequence opens the heart chakra and purifies and balances the sun and moon channels, building wisdom energy.

NIGUMA YOGA SEQUENCE 8
One Leg

Moving in the Sequence

1. Seated in the vajra posture, perform a cycle of arrow breathing and establish a vase breath. Break the posture and stand up quickly.
2. Raise both arms to shoulder height and stretch them out to the sides. Keep the tips of the thumbs at the base of the ring fingers.
3. Lift the right leg up to thigh level, rotate the thigh externally, clockwise, and place the sole of the right foot high upon the left thigh. Take care not to touch the knee. The foot should press into the flesh of the thigh firmly. Depending on your flexibility, the knee will angle out directly to the side or partially, but the pelvis should stay neutral.
4. Hop three times in a steady rhythm while keeping your arms, hands, and lifted leg in the same position.
5. Keeping the arms lifted in the same position, switch legs and hop again three times.

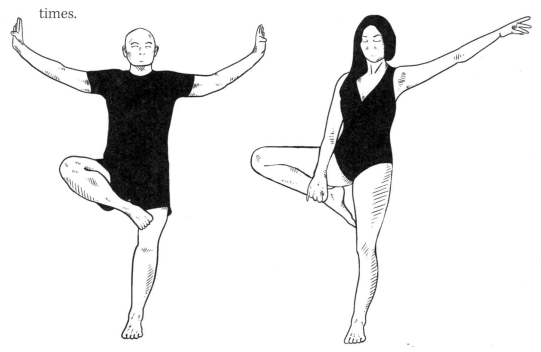

6. Bring both legs to a neutral standing posture. Ensure the vase breath is well established and release the posture to a seat or perform a bep.

7. Hands will land on the knees with open palms and thumbs to ring fingers as you land in the seat and the arrow breath is released.

Precautions and Contraindications

Knee injuries; traumatic brain injuries, vertigo, and poor eyesight limiting balance; and pregnancy for risk of falling.

Precautions and Contraindications

Never place your foot on the knee, but rather press into the thigh flesh.

Benefits

Balance is crucial for brain function, mental focus, ankle stability, promoting postural alignment, core muscles, and strength to the lower body: hip joints, glutes, and legs. Hopping is used in the Niguma yoga system to move the lower winds up and gather energy into the central channel, cultivating bliss and a luminous mind.

Preparations

Practice tree pose at a wall. Extend your arm far toward the wall, with the fingers just barely touching the wall. Find a point to gaze toward on the ground. Single-point earth-gazing like this will help you remain steady in mind and body. Work at cultivating stability through grounding the four corners of your feet and drawing up the sheaths of your leg muscles and arches. Open the hips with the figure-four posture (see page 92) and other hip and glute stretches from hatha yoga. Practice tree pose until you have the steadiness and mobility to do the Niguma yoga hop with breath retention.

Practice warrior poses from hatha yoga to gain external hip rotation mobility and leg strength. Practice gazing the eyes at a single point in standing poses like warrior 2 to cultivate steadiness and balance in the physical body and mind. Open the hips in externally rotated seated poses like janu sirsasana and baddha konasana (bound angle pose; see page 93).

NIGUMA YOGA SEQUENCE 9
Two Legs

Moving in the Sequence

1. Seated in the vajra posture, perform a cycle of arrow breathing and establish a vase breath.
2. Break the posture and stand up quickly.
3. Stretch out the right leg and arm diagonally in front of the body to around 2 o'clock.
4. Simultaneously turn the arm and leg counterclockwise in a generous circle three times, like you are stirring a pot.
5. Quickly reverse the rotation and land the lifted foot back on the ground next to the other foot. At the same time, the arm circles back one time, and as the foot lands, the hand also lands on the outer thigh with a gentle slap.
6. Repeat the sequence with the left arm and leg: circle three times counterclockwise and then once back, with the hand slapping the outer thigh and foot landing in a neutral stance.
7. From this neutral standing position, ensure the vase breath is strongly established and release the posture with the classic hand break posture, then take a seat or perform a bep.
8. Finish the posture in the seated vajra posture and complete the arrow breath. As the breath finishes, the hands land on the knees with fingers extending outward. The thumbs stay pressed to the base of the ring fingers.
9. Focus on the bottom of the exhalation to calm the mind and meditate on the mind's luminosity.

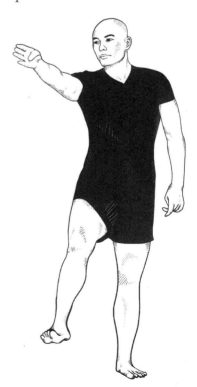

Precautions and Contraindications
Traumatic brain injuries, vertigo, and risk of falling.

Preparations
Hip mobility and balance poses.

Subtle Body Highlights
This sequence opens and clears the base chakra and channels, and gathers the wind energies.

NIGUMA YOGA SEQUENCE 10

Twisting

Moving in the Sequence

1. Seated in the vajra posture, perform a cycle of arrow breathing and establish a vase breath.
2. Break the posture and stand up quickly.
3. Slide your hands up the side of the body to chest level, then hook your thumbs inside your armpits while interlocking your fingers tightly at the center of your chest. Keep your arms and elbows level with the shoulders in a straight line.
4. Take a deep lateral bend to the right, then come back up and lateral bend to the left, and then move back to the right again and finish back at center. Feel the stretch from the head down to the side of the hips. Keep your head neutral with a forward gaze and avoid bending forward or backward. In this way, stretch the right side twice and the left just once.

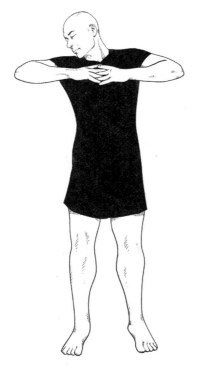
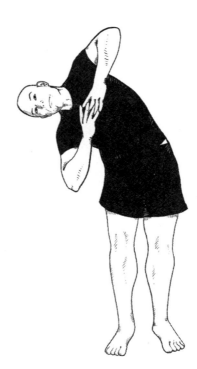

5. Keeping your hands and arms just as they are, take a cross-legged seat. No bep is performed.
6. Once seated, take a lateral bend to the right, then left, then back to the right, just as you did while standing.
7. Shift your body weight forward toward your knees and make your hands into vajra fists.
8. Bring the left arm and fist in front, with the fist in front of the heart, and bring the right vajra fist behind the back to heart level.

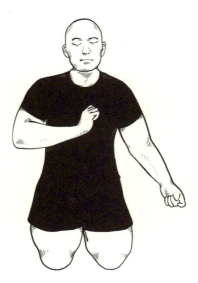

9. Prepare to jump and turn the body to the left from front facing to backward facing. Gather momentum by quickly swinging your arms and torso to the right and then use the edges of your feet to lift your seat off the ground and gain momentum to jump and twist to the left, turning the body 180 degrees to land in a kneeling position. As you land, the vajra fists switch, so that the right fist is now in front of the heart and the left fist is to the back.
10. Quickly reverse the movement and hop back to front, again landing on your knees and switching the vajra fists.
11. Finally, quickly hop from your knees back to a cross-legged seat with your hands striking the knees as you land. The arrow breath is then released as you open your hands and extend the fingers. Take three calming breaths and

focus on the pause at the bottom of your exhalation, cultivating the mind's luminosity.

Precautions and Contraindications

Knee surgery that does not allow for full knee closure upon kneeling and if you are experiencing pain. Avoid if there is bone-on-bone osteoarthritis or knee pain upon kneeling, lumbar ligament strain, or pain upon side bending.

Preparations

Lateral bends with hands clasped over the head to maximize extension of the side body. Virasana and child's pose to gain flexibility kneeling. After a knee surgery, if the knee joint doesn't close, use wooden rods or wool blankets wedged tight at the knee creases to give support and fill any excess space behind the knee.

Subtle Body Highlights

Side bending clears and opens the sun and moon channels. Once the prana vital wind energy is moving freely, the yogi can then begin to direct the flow of energy into the central channel. As the lateral body and intercostal muscles of the ribs open in side bending, one's lung capacity increases, and in turn the wind energies can freely flow. Mind and breath, called chitta *and* prana *in Sanskrit, move together and become expansive. Any blockages—called* samskaras, *which are mental patterns and addictions—that have been imprinted in the side channels are given the opportunity to clear from this bending and twisting practice, and one can recognize the boundless and luminous original nature of being.*

NIGUMA YOGA SEQUENCE 10 SUPPORTING PRACTICES

Side bending benefits the physical and subtle body greatly. It increases our lung capacity by opening up and strengthening the intercostal muscles, the muscles between the ribs. Side bending stretches the arms, shoulders, torso, and lower back, and it improves tight hips and the band of muscle and fascia on the outside of the leg.

Niguma postures 10, 17, 19, and 21 utilize strong lateral bending. In all of these sequences, the arms are folded in some way, which requires you to utilize your core because both arms are positioned close to the body. This arm folding also can make it more difficult to get the extension needed to make your lower back feels good in the pose. Until your core is strong enough to support a hands-free posture, work with the following postures that utilize the ground or extended arms to support the back.

Seated Crescent Pose

Moving into the Pose
1. Take a cross-legged seat, kneel, or sit at the edge of a chair.
2. Press down to the earth with the pelvis or legs and elongate your spine.
3. Place your left hand to the side of your left hip so you can ground down and leverage more spinal extension, and then lift the torso up away from the ground. You can also place your left hand on a block.
4. Inhale, lift the pit of the abdomen toward the navel, and reach your right arm overhead. Rotate the right arm internally so the palm faces in and the shoulder blade can move out toward the side of the body.
5. Keep reaching the arm higher, and then begin to bend to your left side. Try not to move forward or backward.

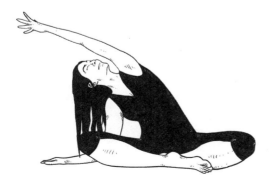

6. Breathe deeply. You are welcome to sway gently in and out of the bend at first to ease into the pose until you find the sweet spot to then hold.

Standing Crescent Moon Pose

Moving into the Pose

1. Stand in mountain pose (tadasana) with feet hip-width apart, or if possible, with feet and thighs together in equal stance pose (samasthiti).
2. Root down through your feet and draw up your arches, leg muscles, lower belly, and pelvic floor. Grounding, or rooting down toward the earth to rise up, activates the muscles at the center of the pelvic floor, and this activation travels on up from the pelvic basin to all of the muscles above, bringing structural integrity throughout the body, space in your discs, length in your muscles, and stability to your joints.
3. Inhale and reach your arms over your head. Interlace your fingers while reaching out through pointed index fingers to emphasize lengthening the body and getting more connected to your core.
4. Keeping the activity in your legs, inhale and lengthen through the arms and side body, and on an exhalation, bend to the right side without leaning forward or back.
5. Take at least five breaths and change sides.
6. If bending with both arms over your head is too much, you can keep one arm by your side or continue to work with the seated side bend with your bottom arm supporting you on the ground.

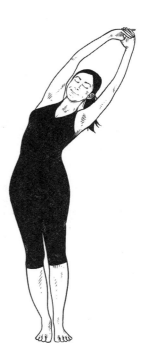

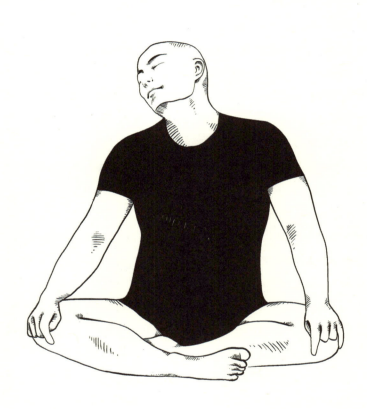

NIGUMA YOGA SEQUENCE 11

Like a Small Child

Moving in the Sequence

1. Seated in the vajra posture, perform a cycle of arrow breathing and establish a vase breath.
2. Break the posture and stay seated with loosely crossed legs and loose vajra fists.
3. Close your eyes. Rotate the head in smooth circles to the right three times, making full head rolls in a clockwise direction.
4. After the head rolls, open your eyes and stand up.
5. Once standing and stable, close your eyes and roll the head three times in each direction.
6. Upon finishing the rotations, open your eyes.
7. From this neutral standing position, ensure the vase breath is strongly established and release the posture with the classic hand break movement, then take a gentle seat. No bep is performed.
8. Finish the sequence in the seated vajra posture and complete the arrow breath. As the breath finishes, the hands land on the knees with fingers extending outward. The thumbs stay pressed to the base of the ring fingers.
9. Focus on the bottom of the exhalation to calm the mind and meditate on the mind's luminosity.

Precautions and Contraindications

Cervical spine injuries, disc herniations, traumatic brain injury, and vertigo.

Preparations

Slow, gentle neck stretches.

Subtle Body Highlights

This sequence opens and clears the throat chakra and purifies and illuminates udana vayu vital wind energy in the throat.

NIGUMA YOGA SEQUENCE 12

Falling

Moving in the Sequence

1. Seated in the vajra posture, perform a cycle of arrow breathing and establish a vase breath.
2. Break the posture and stand up quickly.
3. Keeping your arms by your sides with loose vajra fists, perform three heel raises and drops.
4. Quickly raise your arms up to chest height and tap the chest with your vajra fists by the pecs.
5. Extend your arms out laterally so the arms are slightly raised to about shoulder level, rather than parallel to one another. Your palms face out with the fingers raised up, while the thumbs stay at the base of the ring fingers.
6. Keeping the arms in this raised "T" position, ensure the vase breath is well established and perform a bep; fall or sit gently into the cross-legged position.
7. Stand up quickly and perform the same sequence again twice more, for a total of three rounds.

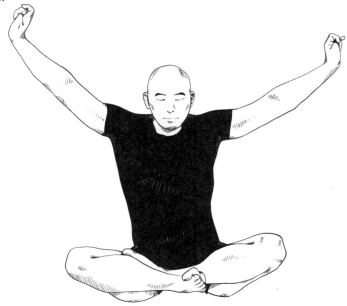

8. Upon the third and final round, the vase breath is released in the seated vajra posture with an arrow breath. As the breath finishes, the hands land on the knees with fingers extending outward. The thumbs stay pressed to the base of the ring fingers.

9. Calm the mind and body by focusing on the bottom of the exhalation and meditate on the mind's luminosity.

Preparations
Deep hip opening, leg strengthening in standing hatha poses, squats, and lunges.

Precautions and Contraindications
Knee or hip injuries, such as meniscus strains or labrum tears; high blood pressure, lumbar disc injuries, and osteoarthritis.

Subtle Body Highlights
This sequence builds heat and adrenaline and drives the winds toward the central channel (uma) to increase bliss.

NIGUMA YOGA SEQUENCE 12 SUPPORTING PRACTICES

HIP OPENING POSTURES

If one is to progress toward performing a full bep, as is done in Niguma yoga sequence 12, the hips must be open enough to land on the ground with the upper and lower thighs evenly striking. This takes consistent hip opening.

Hip mobility and strength is not only important for gaining the ability to perform the Niguma yoga postures; it also is essential for our general well-being and longevity. Tight and immobile hips contribute to knee injuries, lower back pain, balance issues, and more. Consistent practice of the following stretches will help you build your vajra posture, also known as lotus posture or padmasana, and a more comfortable crossed-legged meditation pose. See the appendix for detailed instructions on getting into the vajra posture and more hip opening postures.

Understand that due to each person's unique physiology, some of us will have the ability to fold our legs into the vajra posture, and some of us will not. Those of us who have narrow hip sockets or bones shaped as such that the femur (thigh bone) can't make the external rotation needed to fold into the pose will need patience and acceptance. You may find that over time it becomes clear that the body's bony structures limit movement into the pose. The limitation comes from the shape and size of the femur and the hip socket (called the acetabulum). If the thigh bone doesn't have room to make the external rotation and hits the pelvis bone, this bone-to-bone contact puts the brakes on further movement. If we don't honor that anatomical structural limitation and try to force our leg into lotus posture, our dear knees can become injured, as they twist out of alignment to force the move when they shouldn't. This can result in meniscus or ligament strain or tears. Even the slightest twinge in the knee is a warning that you have gone too far. Great awareness, patience, and compassion is needed as we practice to ensure we honor the precious gift that is our body.

For those who are stiff, in some ways that can be a blessing. The sensation of that stiffness or any other obstacles you have in your yoga practice can actually be transformative. The limitations and sensations felt in the stiffness become a portal for meditative insight, wisdom, and compassion, as these obstacles are an opportunity to practice patience, slow down, and be mindful of the body. Please be careful and practice patiently and consistently.

Figure Four Pose

Figure four pose is one of the best practices for beginners and for opening tight outer hip muscles. It can be done lying down, leaning back while seated, lying down with legs up on a wall, standing with one leg on a desk, or in a seated forward fold known as fire log or double pigeon. Whichever form your pose takes, the most important technique is to keep the foot of the leg you are stretching in a dorsal flexed position, meaning the toes are curled back actively toward the top of the foot. Because the knee joint is open, a dorsal flexed foot will keep the stretch in your hip and not in your knee. The foot is best aligned in the same plane as the shin, positioned as it is when you are standing. If you have an open wall space, you can practice a variation of this pose with the legs up the wall, which will allow you to spend more time in the pose and relax into a longer held stretch.

Figure Four Pose at a Wall

Moving into the Pose

1. Lie down with your legs up a wall and pelvis neutral. Bend your right leg and place the ankle on top of the left thigh, not on the knee.
2 If your pelvis is tipping back, slide away from the wall until it can rest in a neutral position.
3. Dorsiflex your feet, such that the toes are curled back actively toward the top of the foot.

4. Slowly bend the leg that is straight up the wall and drag the heel down to where you get the best stretch, without allowing your pelvis to lift off the floor or rotate.
5. Be mindfully aware of the sensation of stretching you are feeling in your leg and breathe with awareness. Stay at least five breaths, twenty seconds or longer.
6. With consistent practice you will build flexibility. Additionally, you can place the foot lower and lower toward the upper thigh and groin to gain further ease in the half-lotus pose.

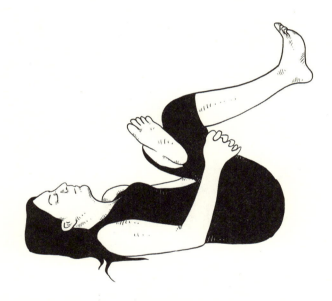

Baddha Konasana (Bound Angle Pose)

Moving into the Pose

1. From a seated posture with legs outstretched (*dandasana* pose), bend the knees and bring the soles of the feet together close to the perineum.
2. Sit at the front edge of your sitting bones. With your fingertips behind you, lift and lengthen the spine. Find an anterior tilt to the pelvis and draw the sacrum into the body. Keeping the anterior tilt to the pelvis, lightly weight the sitting bones toward the earth and recoil the perineum upwards.

3. Hold onto the feet. Press the feet together to open the groin. Press out from the hips to the knees to externally rotate the thigh bones and bring the knees closer to the floor.
4. Inhale and open the heart; on the exhalation, move into the pose with a straight spine and the softest groin possible.
5. Open the soles of the feet like you are opening a book, and if you can keep the spine straight at least half-way down, move further into the pose to ultimately bring the chin to the floor. The opening of the feet will facilitate the full external rotation of the femur bones in the hip socket. Avoid holding the feet closed, as this can strain the knee.
6. Stay in the pose at least five breaths and then inhale, lifting the spine straight, and exhale to rise up. Place your hands under the knees to support yourself while lifting out of the pose.

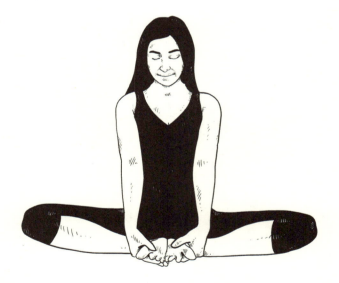

Prop Work

If you are stiff and your back is rounding and your pelvis is tilting backward when attempting this pose, the use of the various props below will assist you in sitting straight to protect your lower back.

- *Sit up on a bolster, block, or folded blankets to assist the anterior tilt of pelvis.*

- *Sit on the ground and place the feet on a block to bring more stretch to the inner thighs.*
- *Sit with your back to the wall to avoid rounding your spine and tilting your pelvis posteriorly.*

Benefits

The bound angle pose stretches the adductor muscles of the inner thighs and opens the hips. It also assists in reproductive health and builds flexibility for other poses central to Niguma yoga, including lotus/vajra posture, beps, and Niguma sequence 22.

NIGUMA YOGA SEQUENCES 13 AND 14
Opening the Uma

Note: Niguma yoga sequences 13 and 14 are practiced together as one seamless sequence.

Moving in Sequence 13

1. Seated in the vajra posture, perform a cycle of arrow breathing and establish a vase breath. Do not break the posture this time.
2. Raise the arms out to the sides to shoulder height, keeping the hands in vajra fists. Look to the right and bend the right arm while keeping the left arm out in a straight line. Strike the right outer chest (pectoralis minor area) with the right vajra fist, then quickly throw the right arm straight out to the right. As your right arm straightens, your left arm bends and strikes the left outer chest. Quickly alternate like this for three rounds, ending with your right arm stretched out to the side and your left arm bent, vajra fist hitting pec.

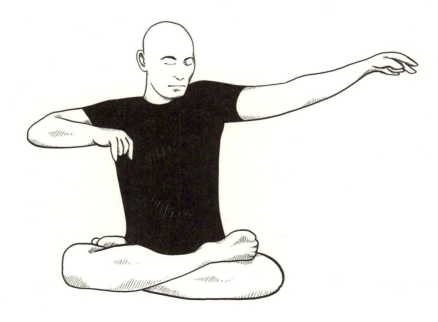

3. Quickly look left and repeat these movements on the left side. The left arm stays bent at the start and strikes the left side of the chest again to begin the sequence for a total of three rounds on the left side.
4. Finish by placing the hands on the knees and release the vase breath. Immediately establish another vase breath for sequence 14.

Moving in Sequence 14
1. While keeping the new vase breath, break the posture and stand up at the back corner of your mat.
2. Bring your hands up by your ears with open palms and thumbs touching the base of the ring fingers. Keep your arms bent, like a tiger getting ready to pounce. The bent arm position also looks like a goal post or cactus.
3. Crouch low and keep your gaze up as you launch your body forward and land on your belly. Your head and legs are up so that you land on your belly with a backbend extension, like a locust pose or flying superhero form. Your arms stay bent in the cactus arm shape.
4. Then place your hands on the ground to push your body up quickly and jump to a cross-legged seat.
5. This all happens in one smooth, quick movement, and finishes as the legs cross and your hands land on the knees to release the arrow breath.

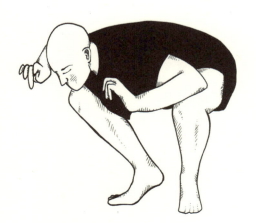
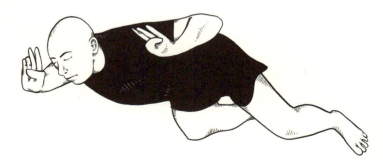

Contraindications

Abdominal hernias, disc injuries, lumbar ligament strain, rotator cuff tears, and pregnancy.

Preparations

From hatha yoga, back extensions such as locust pose and cobra will assist in your ability to perform this sequence. Pushups will build controlled arm strength. Contra lateral back strengthening leg raises will build core and back strength. Kneeling opposite arm-leg extensions and opposite arm-leg extensions performed on the belly will also help prepare for this sequence.

Subtle Body Highlights

These two sequences increase bliss, as the prana vital wind energy from the heart is stimulated with the chest strikes and directed toward the navel, and the samana vital wind energy at the navel is stimulated when landing on the belly. The kurma vital wind energy in the rear channels and vyana vital wind energy both govern the extension and contraction of the limbs. Vyana energy governs the water element and flows from the heart throughout the body into the periphery, similar to the vagus nerve. Samana vital wind energy is associated with the wind element, and when opened, it is said kundalini rises or chandali fire is built. As one drops back to a seat, the landing invites the central channel (uma) to further open and receive the awakened energy.

NIGUMA YOGA SEQUENCE 14 SUPPORTING PRACTICES
Building the Core and Back Extension

Building deep core and back extensor strength is helpful for all meditators who spend long periods of time sitting, and regular practice of these poses counteracts the excessive back rounding and weakness that results from a modern lifestyle. These postures keep the discs in the spine healthy and even aid in recovery after back injury. Contralateral actions, like the first exercise here, are particularly safe and therapeutic. Alignment in back extension and core poses will build the awareness and strength needed for performing various Niguma yoga sequences, including 14, where you jump onto the belly and quickly pick up the arms and legs, and 22, in which you perform a sit-up action on the back.

Opposite Arm-Leg Extension

Moving into the Pose

1. Come to your hands and knees, with the knees directly under your hips and hands stacked under your shoulders.
2. Press down into the earth, grounding evenly through your hands and feet, and draw up the lower belly. Isometrically pull your knees and hands toward each other to feel your oblique muscles activate.
3. Keeping your right hand rooted, extend your right leg straight back and place the right foot's toes on the ground.

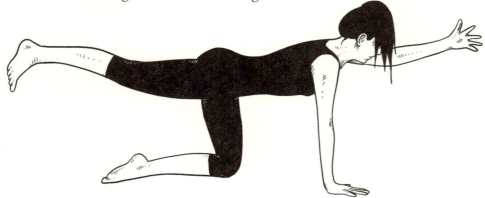

4. Internally rotate the right leg and press the inner heel toward the sky while firming the leg muscles into the bones.
5. Keeping an inner spin to the leg, extend through the toes and lift it to the sky in line with the spine.
6. Now try extending the left arm into the air with the palm turned in.
7. Hold for five to ten breaths and then switch sides.

Benefits
Strengthens back extensors, multifidi (the deep muscles along the spine), quadratus lumborum (the deepest abdominal muscles that support the lower back and extend from the last rib to the pelvis), transversus abdominis (front and side abdominal wall muscles that provide thoracic and pelvic stability), and a symphony of core muscles, as well as the glutes.

Shalabhasana (Locust Pose)

Moving into the Pose
1. Lie on your stomach with your arms along the side of your body.
2. If your shoulders are tight, turn your palms up. Otherwise you can keep the palms pressing into the ground.
3. Internally rotate both legs without turning your knees in and widen your upper thighs to create space in your lower back.
4. Take a deep inhalation and set your shoulders onto the back by activating the muscles between your shoulder blades and lifting the top of the arm bones toward the sky.

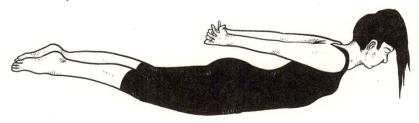

5. Exhale and tone the pelvic floor, draw up the pit of the abdomen, and tone the buttocks. Empty of breath, begin to powerfully contract your hamstrings and move the legs and torso into extension and up off the ground. Inhale after starting the lift.

5. Breathe and keep lengthening out and up while continuing to draw your shoulders onto the back.

6. Exhale down and rest folded hands under your forehead, breathing into your back.

Variations

Hands clasped as shown here to support more chest and shoulder opening; backs of hands to ground and elbows slightly bent to reduce overextending if your back pinches; arms lifting palms up to strengthen the upper back and shoulders; arms above head, superhero style, to increase difficulty and further build your core. Table-top contralateral extensions, using the opposite arm-leg on hands and knees, is helpful to start with if there is pinching in the back.

NIGUMA YOGA SEQUENCE 15
Entering the Uma

Moving in the Sequence

1. Seated in the vajra posture, perform a cycle of arrow breathing and establish a vase breath.
2. Break the posture and stand up quickly.
3. Extend both arms straight out in front of your shoulders and parallel to each other and the ground, with the hands in vajra fists.
4. Keeping the arms shoulder height, bend the elbows, strike the pectoralis with the fist, and then snap the elbows into the side body quickly. Thrust the arms straight in front again and repeat the sequence twice more, for a total of three rounds.

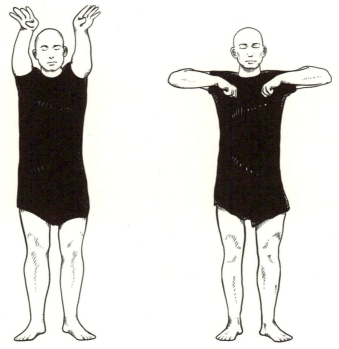

5. Finish by lowering the arms along the side body. Perform three heel raises and drops.

6. Sweep loose vajra fists up the side of the body to shoulder height and then extend the arms out laterally to a make a T at shoulder height. Open the palms out while keeping the thumbs to the base of ring fingers. The fingers point up.

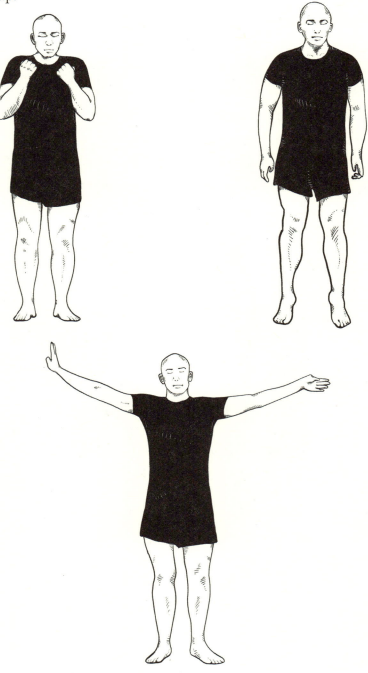

7. Then, keeping the T, swing your body to the right. The left arm will swing forward and the right will swing back. This swing gathers momentum to then strongly swing back to the left, counterclockwise. Then, make a motion like swinging an axe over your head to chop wood, raise the arms up over the left shoulder and overhead, and then throw them down toward the ground in front of you. As the arms come down, strongly exhale with a *ha* breath (an open mouth exhalation that makes the sound "ha!") and shake the shoulders and arms, moving any stuck energy and releasing any negative energy or obscurations.

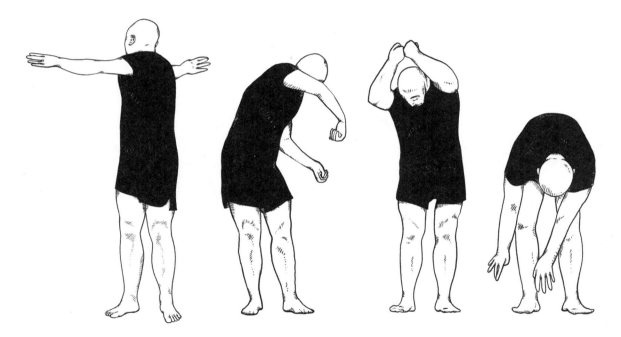

8. Then, begin to raise up again with an inhalation, swinging the arms over the left shoulder, and when they come back down toward the ground, shake them strongly. Repeat this movement three times with *ha* breath exhalations.
9. Return to the vajra posture by simply taking a seat. Focus on the bliss at your center and your mind's luminous original and expansive nature.

Precautions and Contraindications
Avoid if there are active rotator cuff shoulder injuries, and move cautiously if you have lumbar strains or disc injuries.

Preparations
Shoulder opening poses, twists, and forward folds.

Subtle Body Highlights
The striking of the chest further awakens prana vital wind energy at the heart. The swinging of the arms above the head opens the crown chakra. The ha *breath and shaking the heart and shoulders moves stuck energy and spreads the vital drops (thigle) throughout the 7,200 channels with an invitation to enter the central channel.*

NIGUMA YOGA SEQUENCE 16
Drawing Up the Uma

Moving in the Sequence

1. Seated in the vajra posture, perform a cycle of arrow breathing and establish a vase breath.
2. Break the posture and stand up quickly.
3. Keeping the hands in vajra fists, fold the arms across the chest with the right on top and place the fists in the armpits. Bring the elbows down to the chest and press the arms into the torso.

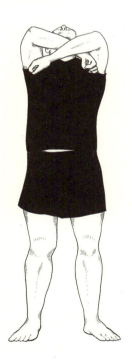 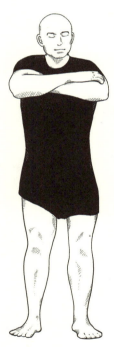

4. With this arm position, bend the torso deeply to the right, then bend to the left, bend forward, and then back. The side bending isn't a straight lateral bend; it is more of a lean into a side bending fold. The head leads the action and moves in the direction you are heading.

5. After leaning back, the arms release along the sides. Ensuring the vase breath is strongly established, release the posture with the classic hand break posture and have a seat or perform a standing bep.

6. Finish the posture in the seated vajra posture and complete the arrow breath. As the breath finishes, the hands land on the knees with fingers extending outward. The thumbs stay pressed to the base of the ring fingers.

7. Focus on the bottom of the exhalation to calm the mind, and meditate on the mind's luminosity.

Contraindications

Lumbar ligament strains, disc injuries, sacroiliac joint pain, and sacral instability.

Preparations

Sun salutations from hatha yoga, lateral bending, back bending, and forward bending.

Subtle Body Highlights

Each bend into the four directions purifies the 7,200 subtle body channels and increases the vital wind energies, such as udana vayu in the front of the body and kurma vayu in the back body. All ten vayus are invited to intensify and flow, which balances the elements the body is made of, and we direct the prana winds to the middle of the body. The bep strike invites the winds to draw up into the central channel (uma) so that one enters timelessness and clarity.

NIGUMA YOGA SEQUENCE 17

Gathering into the Uma 2

Moving in the Sequence

1. Seated in the vajra posture, perform a cycle of arrow breathing and establish a vase breath.
2. Break the posture and stand up quickly.
3. Cross the arms over your chest, placing the right forearm on top of the left. Your hands clasp the opposite arm just above the elbow. Your elbows rest close to the torso.
4. With this arm position, and while holding the vase breath, swirl the hips and the belly in a hula hoop motion three times counterclockwise and three times clockwise.
5. Then, lateral bend to the right, to the left, and then to the right again.

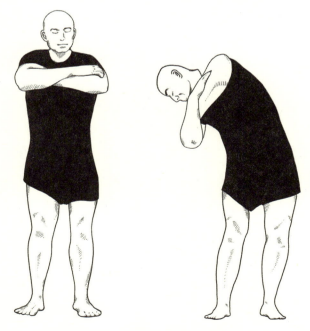

6. Once centered, move the hands from the arms up in a sweeping circular movement to rest the arms and hands by your sides.

7. Sit down gently.
8. Once your seat is established, take your vajra fists to your knees and release the vase breath with an arrow breath and extend the fingers.
9. Calmly breathe and meditate on the luminous nature of being.

Precautions and Contraindications
Avoid if lumbar ligament or intercostal muscle strains or herniated discs are actively present, and move slowly if you have a history of back pain.

Preparations
Lateral bending in hatha yoga. Sufi grinds from kundalini yoga.

Subtle Body Highlights
The churning and circling of the pelvis accompanied by a held vase breath gathers the winds at the base of the central channel and transforms them into wisdom energy to be brought into the central channel. The side bending pours the sun and moon channels together, creating a state of equanimity and balanced wind energy flow.

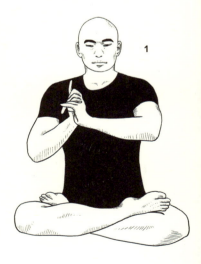

1

NIGUMA YOGA SEQUENCE 18
Yoga Practice that Dispels the Kleshas (Addictions)

This sequence consists of three parts that can be performed separately, using three separate vase breaths, or done sequentially with one vase breath.

18a: Dispelling Ignorance with the Mudra of Buddha Vairochana

Part 1

1. Seated in the vajra posture, perform a cycle of arrow breathing and establish a vase breath. Do not break the posture.
2. Stretch the arms forward and place the left index finger in the center of the right palm and wrap the fingers of the right hand around it, with the right index finger extended.
3. Strike the right outer pec near the shoulder with this mudra once, then strike the left, then the lower abdomen, then the middle of the chest.

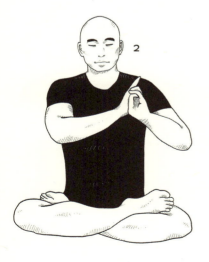 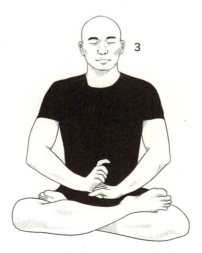 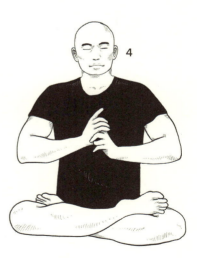

Part 2

1. Immediately bring both arms forward and stretch out the hands and fingers with open palms.
2. Part the hands in a swimming/sweeping action, then bring the hands back to slap the outer thighs.
3. When striking the thighs, lean forward to lift the buttocks off the floor, then rock back to a seat and repeat. Perform this breaststroke-like action with the arms in coordination with the seat lifts three times in total.

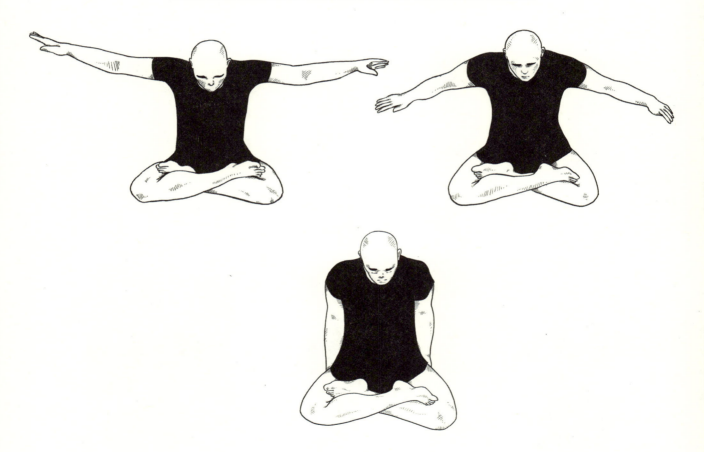

18b: Dispelling Irritation

Part 3

1. Turn the left palm up like you are holding water in your palm at a level four finger-widths below the navel, like the hand mudra of Amitabha Buddha; turn the right palm in at the heart level in a one-handed prayer position, like the mudra of Buddha Amoghasiddhi. See the image of Rinpoche below for clarity on the hand mudras.
2. Simultaneously strike the chest and the lower abdomen with these mudras three times quickly and firmly.
3. Finish the posture in the seated vajra posture and complete the arrow breath. As the breath finishes, the hands land on the knees with fingers extending outward. The thumbs stay pressed to the base of the ring fingers.

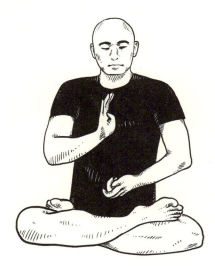

Subtle Body Highlights

The Sanskrit word klesha *has been translated variously as poison, obscuration, hindrance, and addiction. The Buddha pointed to there being five primary kleshas: ignorance, aversion/hatred, craving/desire, pride, and jealousy. In Vajrayana Buddhism these are to be transformed into wisdom energy rather than things to be transcended, as in other traditions. The presence of these addictions creates blockages in our energy channels, with ignorance known as the major obstacle to the central channel opening, anger blocking the sun channel on the right, and desire blocking the moon channel on the left. Prana, in the form of the most refined and subtle breath, is connected to the highest form of awakened luminous mind. Enlightenment is said to correspond to knowing that reality is bliss that realizes emptiness, and it can be directly experienced as the wind energies flow freely throughout all 7,200 channels and enter into the central channel. The hand gestures, or mudras, in this series strike the right, left, and central channels, and are the symbols of the buddhas that have transformed these once-poisons into intuitive wisdom (jnana) and the nectar of immortality (amrita). The first sequence is devoted to the buddha Vairochana, who transforms ignorance into primordial wisdom. The second sequence, with the hands striking the outer thighs, is devoted to buddhas Akshobhya and Ratnasambhava, who transform anger into mirror-like wisdom and pride into equality wisdom. The last is devoted to buddhas Amitabha and Amoghasiddhi, who transform desire into discriminating wisdom and jealousy into all-accomplishing wisdom.*

NIGUMA YOGA SEQUENCE 19
Dispelling Agitation

Moving in the Sequence

1. Seated in the vajra posture, perform a cycle of arrow breathing and establish a vase breath. Do not break the posture.
2. Interlace the fingers with the pinky fingers remaining separate. Intertwine the ring fingers.
3. Place this mudra at the back of your neck with the pinky side of the hand resting at the base of the head and the ring fingers extending down to touch the bottom of the neck at the seventh vertebra.

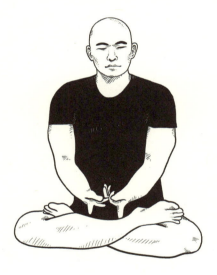 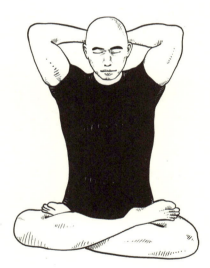

4. Keeping the mudra resting on the neck, lean the body deeply to the right, touching the elbow to the ground if possible, and then return to an upright position with the gaze straight ahead. Then bend deeply to the left and return upright. Then once more bend deeply to the right and return to center. Right, left, right, for a total of three side bends.

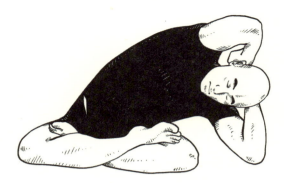

5. Release the hand mudra from behind the head and take the arms down, extending them with hands near knees.
6. Gracefully lift the arms back up and out to the sides at shoulder height.

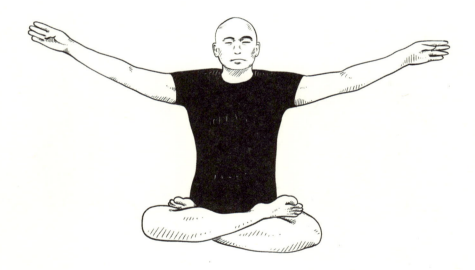

7. With the palms facing inward, bend the arms at the elbows and gently slap or tap the forehead three times while gazing straight ahead and trying not to blink. The eyes should stay wide open, gazing forward just above the horizon line.
8. Bring the arms back down, extending them with vajra fists at the knees, and complete the arrow breath.
9. Abide in spacious awareness.

THE YOGA OF NIGUMA SEQUENCES: ILLUSTRATIONS AND INSTRUCTIONS   117

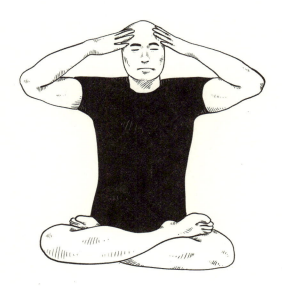

Preparations
Lateral bending, chest and arm opening stretches, and neck stretches. Trataka, meaning look or gaze in Sanskrit, is a hatha yogic purification and a tantric method of meditation that involves staring at a single point, such as a candle flame. This is a good preparation for this sequence as it teaches us to gaze with open eyes while not blinking, as is done above. Practicing Buddhist calm-abiding meditation with eyes open is also a wonderful preparation, as it teaches us single-point concentration and to stay undisturbed no matter what is arising. As we slap the forehead with open, unblinking eyes in this sequence, we are demonstrating this steadiness of mind.

Precautions and Contraindications
Avoid if neck, rib, or quadratus lumborum ligament strains are present.

Subtle Body Highlights
Focusing on the right channel while bending twice to that side emphasizes the purification of the klesha, or obscuration, of anger and agitation. Slapping the forehead symbolizes waking up the higher mind (buddhi) that has the faculty of discernment to see reality clearly, in freedom and bliss. Indian inner science says that what is

blocking our intuitive wisdom, or jnana, from shining forth under the light of discriminative awareness is mis-knowing and the templates of belief that keep us repeating patterns that cause suffering. The buddha nature that abides in all of us is illuminated in meditative practices such as those which Niguma has gifted us.

NIGUMA YOGA SEQUENCE 20
Overpowering the Harmful

Moving in the Sequence

1. Seated in the vajra posture, perform a cycle of arrow breathing and establish a vase breath. Do not break the posture.
2. Gracefully extend your arms in front of you and form the blazing mudra with your hands, in which your hands and fingers are spread open with the right thumb resting over the left thumb and the left index finger resting over the right. This creates a triangular window to gaze through. The other fingers fan out so that the window is centered. Your palms face outward.

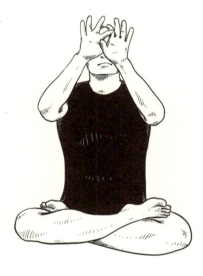

3. Bring the arms over to the right, around 1 o'clock, and while looking meditatively through the space within the window, roll your wrists and move the hands in a wave-like manner four times.
4. Move the hands and gaze to the left side, around 11 o'clock, and repeat four wave-like rolls as you gaze into the space between.
5. Move the hands, gaze to the center and above the brow, and repeat the waves.

6. Move the hands and gaze down in the direction of 6 o'clock and repeat the four waves.

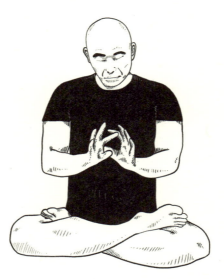

7. Lastly, move the hands straight in front around brow level, so that the gaze is at the level of the horizon, and repeat the four rolling waves.
8. Break the blazing mudra by bringing loose vajra fists back toward one's face with palms facing inward, and sweep down like you are washing the face, but without touching it, and then return the hands to the knees with arms extended.
9. Complete the arrow breath in sync with the hands landing on the knees. Spread the fingers as the arrow lands.

Physical benefits

Improves the accuracy of your memory as you increase the neural activity across the front of the two brain hemispheres.

Subtle Body Highlights

These movements call upon the five wisdom buddhas (dhyani buddhas) in the five directions (the four cardinal directions and center) to help us overcome the five harmful kleshas: ignorance, aversion, desire, pride, and jealousy. The five wisdom buddhas are Vairochana, who transforms ignorance; Akshobhya, who transmutes aversion, which also manifests as anger and aggression; Amitabha, who transforms desire; Ratnasambhava, who transforms pride; and Amoghasiddhi, who transforms jealousy. As we gaze to the five directions we also open our 7,200 channels and balance and increase the wind energy of the five vayus: prana centered in the heart and up, apana below, udana centered above, and vyana to the sides, with samana vayu coming online as the others are united. This balance invites the outer winds' energies to merge together at the central channel. We overpower any harmful obscurations and abide in the freedom, wisdom, and bliss at our center.

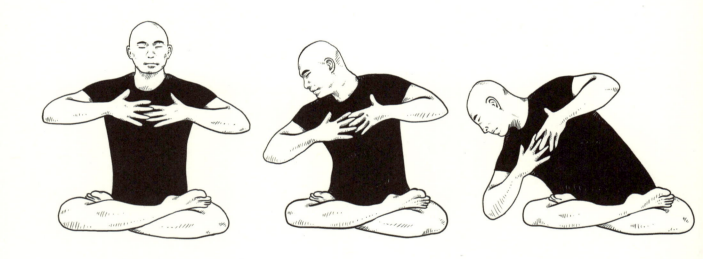

NIGUMA YOGA SEQUENCE 21

Dispelling Aggression and Aversion with the Mudra of Akshobhya and Dispelling Pride with the Mudra of Amitabha

Note: Traditionally this sequence was passed down in the lineage as three parts, but they should be performed sequentially with one vase breath if possible. The vase breath is released with a strong vocal "ha!" sound at the end of the third part.

Moving in the Sequence

1. Seated in the vajra posture, perform a cycle of arrow breathing and establish a vase breath. Do not break the posture.

21a. Dispelling Aggression and Aversion with the Mudra of Akshobhya

2. Place your two open palms over your chest at the heart level. Your fingers touch one another.
3. Keeping the hands like this, with the elbows kept shoulder height out to the sides, side bend to the right while looking down toward the ground that you are leaning toward. Refrain from leaning forward or backward. This is a straight lateral bend. You will side bend to the right three times. Each time, go a little further. There is a slight springing back between each repetition.
4. Repeat another three bends on the left side.

21b. Meditative Gazing

5. Return to center and release the hands in the form of loose vajra fists at the knees.

6. Keeping the arms extended, fists on the knees, and your head upright, smoothly glide your head in a turn to float the gaze to the right above the horizon.

7. Slowly and smoothly glide the head to turn and look to the left, floating the gaze above the horizon.

8. Slowly return the head back to center and gaze straight ahead.

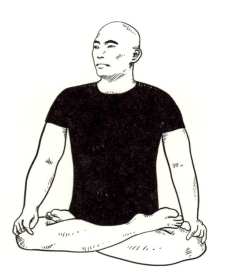 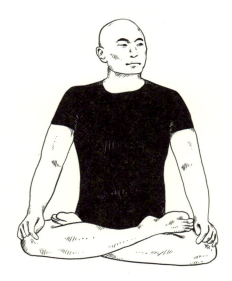

21c. Dispelling Pride with the Mudra of Amitabha

9. Place your hands in the mudra of Buddha Amitabha to dispel pride by first raising the arms out straight in front, slightly above one's eye level, and with palms down.

10. Turn the palms up and place the right hand on top of the left hand, with both palms facing up and thumbs lightly touching, thus making the Amitabha mudra.

11. Use this hand mudra to strike the lower abdomen at a point four finger-widths below the navel three times using the inner edges of the hands. As each strike lands, exhale with a strong "ha!" sound.

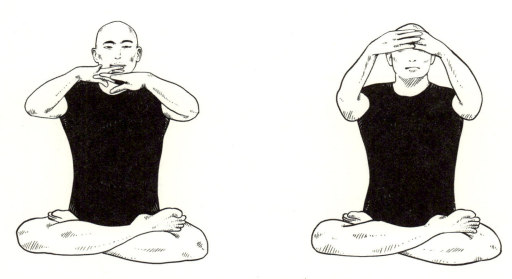

12. Finish the posture by placing the vajra fists on the knees and rest in the vajra posture in meditation.

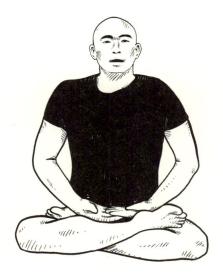

Preliminaries

Supported lateral bends and gentle neck stretches.

Physical Benefits

Aids contralateral hemispheric activation of the brain, memory, and neck mobility, and balances the endocrine system.

Subtle Body Highlights

This sequence aids in the purification and balancing of the sun and moon channels. The klesha of aggression or aversion lives in the sun channel on the right, and pride, which stems from ignorance and clinging to ego, lives in the moon channel on the left side. Hatha yoga and Tibetan yoga practices both purify, balance, and transform these obscurations that get stuck in our channels, thus releasing misperceptions and returning us to our natural state of clarity, bliss, and nondual awareness.

Niguma yoga opens the body's channels, winds, and drops (Skt. nadi, vayu, *and* bindu; *Tib.* tsa, lung, *and* thigle) *as a method of transforming suffering into wisdom and compassion. Side bending opens the sun and moon channels, head turns open the udana vayu in the throat to purify speech, while the strike at the navel and "ha!" breath opens the central channel as it stimulates the samana vayu to transform ignorance into bliss.*

NIGUMA YOGA SEQUENCE 22
Dispelling Desire

Moving in the Sequence

1. Seated in the vajra posture, perform a cycle of arrow breathing and establish a vase breath.
2. Break the posture and lift the right leg approximately four inches off the ground in front of the left, with the right arm hovering around four inches just above it. Both the arm and the leg stay bent.

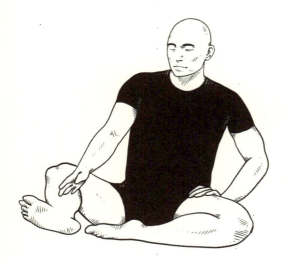
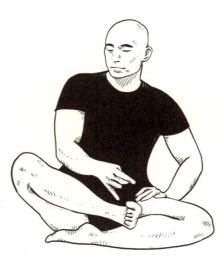

3. Circle the right leg and arm counterclockwise with a stirring-like action. The arm and leg move together as if they were attached, even though they don't touch. The palm is facing down.
4. Circle three times counterclockwise.
5. Switch directions and perform a semicircle back in the clockwise direction, then lay the leg down to rest on the ground in a frog-like position. As the leg hits the ground, the right hand and arm turn palm up and strike down onto the inner leg with a slap.

6. Leaving the right arm and leg in this position, repeat the sequence with the left leg and arm. This time, the circling motions are directed clockwise three times.

7. Finish by circling back once counterclockwise to lay the leg to the ground as the left palm turns up and slaps the inner leg. Now both legs are open in a frog-like position with both arms resting palms facing up.

8. Recline onto the mat with the legs outstretched and lifted off the ground along with the torso, such that only the lower back and pelvis remain touching the ground. This position looks like the hatha yoga posture ardha navasana, or half-boat, sometimes called hollow body. It also looks like you're on a luge sled.

9. Lift your arms above your chest and make a circle with them, bringing the fingers together to touch. It will look like you are holding a full moon in your arms.

10. Keeping this position, pull your right knee toward your chest to bend the leg, and then switch legs to extend right and bend the left. Perform five cycles of pulling in the legs. This is not a bicycle movement but a knee-hip flexion and extension. Take care to keep the lower black flat to the ground.

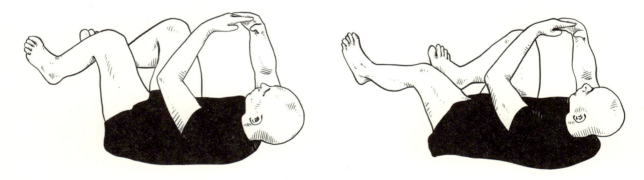

11. Keep the eyes steady in space in the direction of the lifted hands.
12. End the sequence by returning to a relaxed cross-legged seat with hands on knees in vajra fists.

13. Open the fingers in time with the forceful exhalation of an arrow breath. The thumbs always remain on the base of the ring fingers.

14. Meditate on the clarity of mind, breath, and body, and engage in a few rounds of breathing, closing vajra fists while drawing in the breath and extending the hands upon exhaling. Notice the natural gaps between each breath and the accompanying spaciousness and luminosity of awareness.

Preliminaries

Supine leg raises; table top extensions; hatha poses such as baddha konasana and upavishta konasana; the yin pose frog; all hip openers; the half-boat pose ardha navasana; and preliminary abdominal strengthening.

Precautions and Contraindications

Lower back strain is possible if the core muscles aren't strong enough to hold you up. Prepare with feet on the ground instead of the hollow body position with extended legs. Hip flexor or adductor pull is possible if one is not strong enough to lift the legs and stir or extend the legs.

Subtle Body Highlights

This sequence opens and strengthens the lower belly and pelvis region that is connected to the klesha of desire in order to clear such craving. The lower thigle, or drop, that connects to creative energy is activated and a fire is awakened to activate the bliss of pure being. Desire is transformed into the wisdom of discernment, the discriminating awareness that sees emptiness and intimacy in all.

NIGUMA YOGA SEQUENCE 22 SUPPORTING PRACTICES
General Core Strength

Ardha Navasana (Half-Boat Pose and Hollow Body)

Moving into the Pose

1. Lie down on the floor with your legs extended and arms by your side.
2. Exhale and engage your core muscles and inner thighs, pressing your lower back to the floor. The back should be completely flat to the ground.
3. Inhale and lift your torso, arms, and legs off the ground without allowing the lower back to lift.
4. Alternatively, if you don't have the strength to lift the legs, bend the legs and sit up with the feet on the ground, or have one leg bent and extend the other, as shown below.
5. Make sure to keep the head neutral.
6. Hold or do gentle rocking movements or sit ups, five to fifty repetitions.

Benefits

Strengthens rectus abdominis (upper abdominal) muscles, transversus abdominis muscles, obliques, hip flexors, and inner thighs. Improves digestion. Tones digestive organs, kidneys, prostate, and bladder.

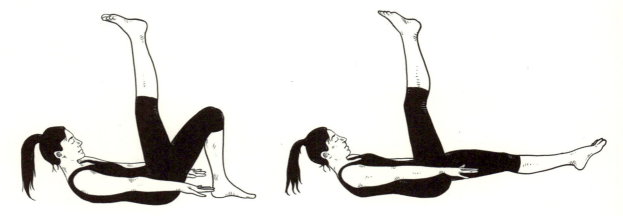

NIGUMA YOGA SEQUENCE 23
The Lesser Descent of Supreme Bliss

Moving in the Sequence

1. Seated in the vajra posture, perform a cycle of arrow breathing and establish a vase breath.
2. Break the posture and remain seated with loosely crossed legs.
3. Lift your arms in front of your chest and turn your left palm up and your right palm down. Hook the right ring finger over the left ring finger and wrap it around tightly so the fingers are locked.
4. Squeeze the chest and upper arms toward the middle and slide your left elbow to the other side of the right elbow. Keep the elbows crossed and ring fingers hooked and thump your left outer shoulder/upper arm with the thumb-side of the right hand. Strike three times quickly. It will make a thumping sound.
5. Release the cross of the arms, flipping the hands over so the right palm is up and the left ring finger hooks over and around the right. The right elbow slides over and across the left. The left hand now strikes the right shoulder three times quickly. Thump using the thumb-side of your left hand.

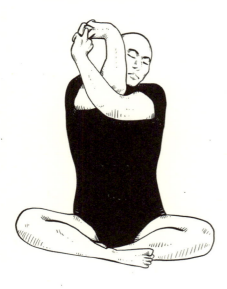
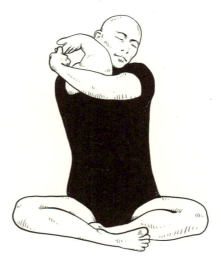

6. End the sequence by returning to a relaxed cross-legged seat with hands on knees in vajra fists. Open the fingers in time with the forceful exhalation of an arrow breath. The thumbs always remain on the base of the ring fingers. Meditate on the clarity of mind, breath, and body. Breathe for a few rounds, closing vajra fists while drawing the breath in and extending the hands upon exhaling. Notice the natural gap between each breath and the accompanying spaciousness and luminosity of awareness.

Preliminaries
Hatha pose garudasana (eagle) and eagle family shoulder opening.

Precautions
Rotator cuff strain is possible if you force the arm across aggressively.

Contraindications
Existing rotator cuff tendon strain or tears, especially involving the infraspinatus tendon.

Subtle Body Highlights
Crossing the midline of the body balances the right and left hemispheres of the brain and pours the right and left channels together to move the wind energy into the central channel, allowing for the descent of supreme bliss.

NIGUMA YOGA SEQUENCE 23 SUPPORTING PRACTICES
Opening the Shoulders

Students often ask what they can do to prepare for the arm action in sequence 23 during in-person teachings. In this posture, the yogi's ring fingers hook and then the chest squeezes together to bring the top arm across until the elbows can stack. Rinpoche often shows a clever method he uses to leverage his arm across: he hooks onto the outside of his lower leg and pushes the top arm across. If you have a lot of muscle like he does, this is a must, as the muscles act as protection for the joints in this movement. This movement is not without risk if you are stiffer or have less stability. For the average person, there is some risk of straining the infraspinatus tendon in the rotator cuff if you use a forceful movement to hook. Nevertheless, we need to cultivate flexibility and range of motion to perform this bind for the health of the shoulder and tendons.

Fortunately, the classic Indian hatha yoga posture named after the mythical eagle-like garuda is a great boon in finding the mobility in the back and shoulders to practice safely and prepare for Niguma yoga sequence 23. The action is the same in both postures.

Garudasana (Eagle Pose)

Moving into the Pose
1. Sit in a cross-legged pose (or stand if you are doing the full pose).
2. Take a deep inhalation and stretch both arms out to the sides to make a T shape.
3. Exhale and swing the right arm under the left, reach out through the arms and fingers to spread the shoulders and upper back, finding as much space as possible.
4. Keeping the shoulders and back spread, try to bring the right forearm on top of the left and bring the palms together.

5. Once the arms are hooked or at their full range of motion, round the back and further spread the shoulder blades like broad eagle wings. Lifting the bound elbows up to at least shoulder height will increase the stretch. Do this gently and continue to breathe into the back and shoulders.

6. Try adding the legs for the full pose, from standing mountain pose with your feet shoulder-width apart, take the right leg over and around the left leg, then hook the right ankle behind the left. Bend the knees and sit back in a chair-like posture, but lift the torso and arms toward the sky. Adding the legs will build leg strength and open the lower back and hips.

Practice the one arm modification as seen below for tight shoulders or when recovering from a rotator cuff tendon injury.

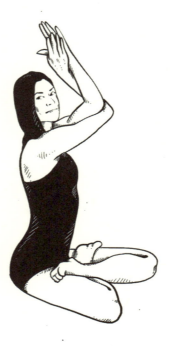
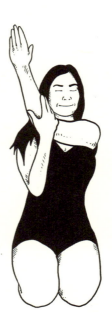

Lying Down Shoulder Stretch

Moving into the Pose

1. Lie down on your belly with your legs outstretched and your hands resting on the ground near your chin.
2. Press your left palm onto the ground and lift the left elbow off the ground, making space to thread the right arm under it.
3. Once the right arm is stretched out to the left, take the left arm over it and reach it out to the right.
4. Pick your torso up and move your body forward so your torso sits over the arms. Use your body weight to spread open the arms and shoulders.
5. Breathe deeply into this intense and very effective shoulder opener.

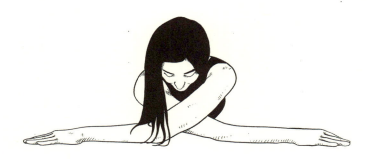

NIGUMA YOGA SEQUENCE 24

The Greater Descent of Supreme Bliss that Dispels Greed

Moving in the Sequence

1. Seated in the vajra posture, perform a cycle of arrow breathing and establish a vase breath.
2. Break the posture and stand up quickly.
3. In a stance with feet hip-width apart, slide the vajra fists up the side of the body to shoulder height and extend them out to the sides. Turn the palms out and keep the thumbs at the base of the ring fingers.

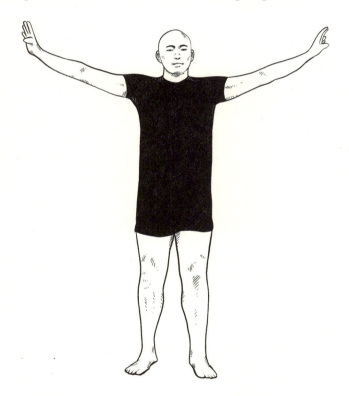

4. Perform three heel raises and drops.
5. Bring the arms back to rest naturally at the sides of the body.

6. Raise an extended right arm with a pointed index finger up the centerline of the body to slightly above shoulder height. Keep your gaze in line with the pointed finger.
7. Then, in a flowing movement, take your right arm and gaze to the right side above the horizon line.
8. Sweep the arm and gaze to the left side.
9. Move the right arm and gaze back to center and straight up toward the sky, then take them down through center to point toward the ground.

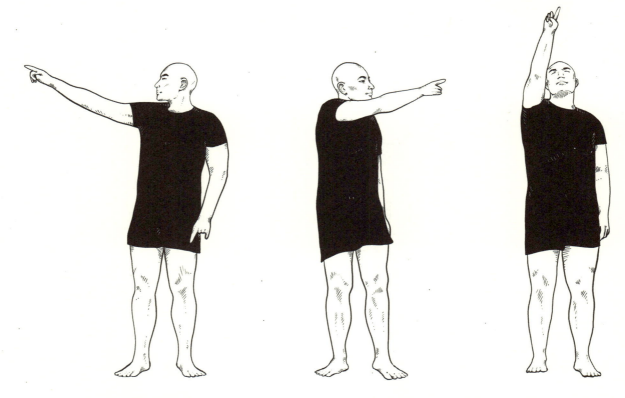

10. Then sweep the right arm and gaze back up so the finger points straight ahead above the horizon line.
11. Keeping the right arm and gaze in this position, now bring up the left arm slightly to the side and then forward to meet the left arm. The two hands will now open and touch each other at the side of the thumbs and index fingers, with the thumb tips moving into the base of the ring fingers.

THE YOGA OF NIGUMA SEQUENCES: ILLUSTRATIONS AND INSTRUCTIONS   139

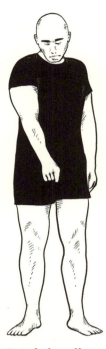
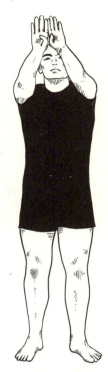

12. Bend the elbows out to the side as you loop the hands back toward your torso. Flip the palms up and glide the hands up the center of the torso to brush against your throat lightly, and then begin to lift them overhead and open them out wide into a backbend, beginning to release the breath with the sound of "haaaahhhh."

13 The *haaaahhhh* breath continues as you lean back into a big back-bending arch, which opens the heart and throat as you sweep the arms up and out wide into a V shape. Keep extending the arms back and down, circle-sweeping them back to your sides. As the arms come back down, the head returns to a neutral position. The *haaaahhhh* breath should end at the same time the arms land back by your sides.

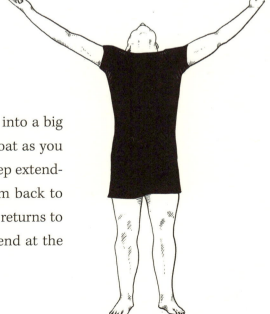

14. Complete the exercise by sitting down gently to a cross-legged seat; there is no bep to fall into the seat. Rest the hands on the knees and observe the expansion into freedom and bliss.

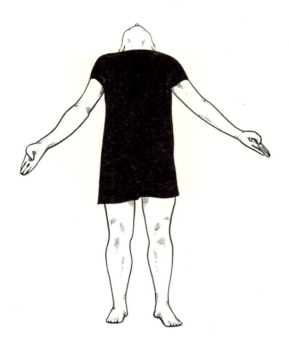

Physical Benefits

Brain health from the controlled eye movements focused down the line of the finger for improved vestibular function and motor coordination; vagus nerve stimulation through the throat opening and vocalization of the breath, as well as the coordinated eye movements; heart opening; shoulder and neck opening; endocrine system balancing.

Precautions and Contraindications

With existing lower back and neck injuries, be cautious of taking too deep of a backbend at the end of this sequence. Try extending up rather than bending back. Avoid dropping the head back if there are disc herniations in the neck. If there is active shoulder joint pain, be cautious of sweeping the arms up overhead until you have healed.

Subtle Body Highlights

The heel drops invite the lower wind energy of apana vayu to move up toward the navel. The gaze to the right and left brings equality to the sun and moon channels and opens the throat and udana vayu. The big back bend and the head turns open the upper winds of prana, vyana, and udana vayu, and pours them back down to meet the lower winds. The meeting of the upper and lower wind energies creates an alchemy that invites heat to rise and supreme bliss to descend. The haaaahhhh *breath spreads the vital essences in the body to increase happiness, well-being, love, wisdom, and compassion.*

NIGUMA YOGA SEQUENCE 25
Shaking "Ha!"

Moving in the Sequence

1. Seated in the vajra posture, perform a cycle of arrow breathing and establish a vase breath. Do not break the posture.
2. Staying seated, make the left hand into a tight vajra fist and bring the arm to the left side of the body. Closely touch the side of the body with the straight left arm and push the vajra fist down into the ground, so the knuckles of the left hand press into the earth.
3. Keeping the arm in that position, make a tight vajra fist with the right hand and use it to vigorously press and sweep down the outside of the left arm three times. Sweep only from the top of the arm to the base of the vajra fist resting on the floor. Each time you bring the right vajra fist back up to the head of the left arm bone it does not touch the arm.

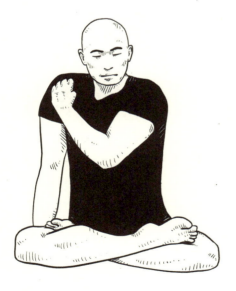 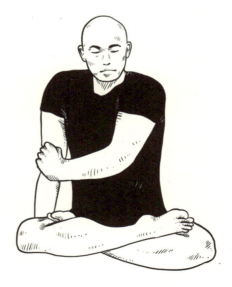

4. Repeat the sequence on the other side.
5. Next, break the posture.

6. Lean forward slightly and use the power in your legs to lift your whole body up and off the ground to perform three small beps. The feet must lift in line with the knees. Practice landing equally on the thighs and buttocks. You should hear a thumping sound upon landing.
7. Next, place open palms on your knees and clutch the knees firmly.
8. Twist the torso to the right side and lean forward while shaking the torso and shoulders as you release the breath with a vocal "ha!" sound.
9. Turn to the left side, lean forward, and shake with the "ha!" sound.
10. Then center the torso and bow forward, toward the ground, and shake with "ha!"
11. End by sitting in the vajra posture or a relaxed cross-legged seat and meditate.

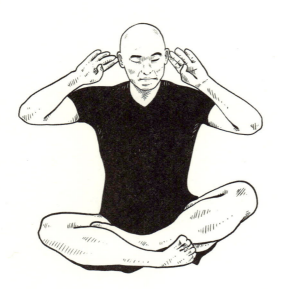
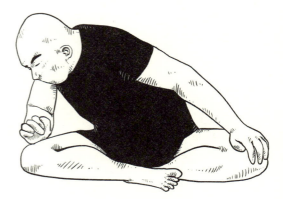

Precautions and Contraindications

When performing small beps, take care to land evenly across the thighs and buttocks with a level pelvis. If you lean too far forward when landing, you can hurt your feet or ankles. If you fall too far back, you can hurt your tailbone (coccyx) or sacrum. Avoid if there are knee injuries, hip injuries, osteoarthritis, or disc injuries.

Preparations

Standing lunges, squats, chair pose, and standing vajra posture can build leg strength to help lift up off the grounds for the small beps. (Vajra posture is the Tibetan yoga pose where the body is shaped in two diamonds, like a vajra, and is performed by turning the feet out, lifting and bringing the heels together, and bending the knees out to the side. The arms are overhead, also in a diamond shape, with the palms together. It can be held for as long as possible.) If you are older and have lost leg and glute strength, standing up and sitting down slowly as you engage your muscles from the edge of a chair with no hands is one of the best ways to build muscle in the legs and is a similar action to lifting up from the ground cross-legged.

Hip openers improve the sitting posture and external rotation of the thighs. If the hips are tight, the knees will not be able to touch the ground in the cross-legged seat. Thus, when landing a bep, you will fall back onto the coccyx. Landing a bep evenly with the front and back of the thigh equally touching the ground is essential, therefore opening the hips so the legs lay flat to the ground when sitting cross-legged is essential. Janu sirsasana (see page 162) can help build the external rotation needed to do this. Yoga mudrasana (cross-legged forward fold) is also very helpful.

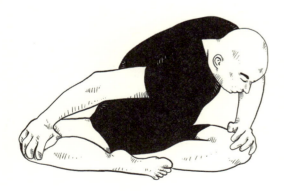
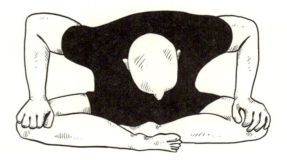

Subtle Body Highlights

The last sequence spreads the vital essence drops throughout the channels. These vital essences first get spread down the channels of the arms. Then the three small beps further invite the subtle body energies that have been gathered and intensified by all the proceeding exercises to move into the central channel and further expand great bliss. Lastly, the shaking in the three directions with the "ha!" breath spreads the vital essence throughout the body, which allows the mind the freedom to abide in happiness and generate wisdom and compassion.

Niguma yoga provides a path to develop a state of well-being that results in an unconditional love that is free from attachment, aversion, and emotions such as pride and jealousy. It increases our wisdom of bliss and emptiness. It keeps the body and mind open and increases our capacity for the most skillful and artful action as we engage with the world and all sentient beings.

6

Conclusion

Each of us is quite fortunate to have the rare opportunity to engage in the practice of the yoga of Niguma. If approached in a safe and careful manner, it is quite accessible and the benefits are many. The yoga of Niguma naturally contributes to and supports one's existing faith by allowing one to experience a deep sense of peacefulness, calm, well-being, and universal connection.

The fruits of the yoga of Niguma illuminated in this book offer the path to great bliss. But these results don't happen by themselves. We must engage and invest ourselves in the practice. The result is not an imaginary promised land but a gradual, profound groundswell of subtle awakening.

There is an initial glimpse of clarity that arises after doing this practice even just for a few days. But with consistent diligence, that seed of clarity sprouts, a sapling grows, and a strong mature tree emerges. At some point, you enter a stage where it is clear that following the path of Dharma leads your mind to expand toward ultimate clarity, compassion, and luminosity.

The essence of this work originated with the Buddha and has manifested over generations. I have attempted to offer these methods and techniques for realization in a manner that best suits the dynamic, and sometimes painful, world of today.

If we truly wish to move beyond the bounds of our mundane state of mind, the principal path follows the teachings of the Buddha. In my experience, there is nowhere else to turn. The Buddha so deeply understood the human condition, and the truth of his teachings still resonates strongly today—the depth of his compassion is still felt and is available to all of us 2,500 years later.

My effort in sharing these teachings with you is simply to share a pristine vehicle so you may achieve a deep joy that is free from suffering, without the burden or distraction of dogma. Dogma leads to blind faith, which too easily results in fixed views that are disconnected from dynamic reality and prevent us from seeing what truly is. The experience of faith is in your own hands, and like any relationship, must continue to be nurtured by returning to the practice again and again. Inevitably, we experience periods of fluidity and progress and then, at other times, we encounter periods where we feel movement to be slow or stuck, even while still practicing. Rather than being too harsh on yourself, strive toward balance. Just ride the waves, release expectations, and let nature take its course.

Hatha yoga, stemming from a different tradition, also has an origin of clarity, but it has become so modernized that too often many of its vast benefits have gone missing from the discourse. There's no benefit to similarly trying to change the yoga of Niguma from its true state or trying to create a new religion or a new form of Buddhism with it. The yoga of Niguma is an ancient, rich practice that comes to us through a pure lineage. It must not be altered or watered down or made into something it is not.

We are all deeply blessed that permissions have been given to teach the yoga of Niguma to the public, but the permissions were given with the proviso that it is taught and practiced truly and properly. In regard to the yoga of Niguma, it has been said that the time for secrets is over. This is because the world is in such a difficult state that the importance of access is now quite vital. Nevertheless, the subtlety and integrity of the practice is fragile and vulnerable. Please understand that what you now have in your hands is most precious. Ultimately, the choice is yours to carry and protect this pristine practice.

Buddhism is all about loving-kindness, sharing happiness, and finding inner peace. It is about being committed to the path of ultimate clarity, engaging with fellow wayfinders, and forging a unity of purpose. The goal of Buddhism is not to convert followers of other faiths.

Rather, Buddhists believe that when misconceptions fall away and the last thin layer of film is removed from one's eyes, all sentient beings naturally reach the clean, clear state of luminosity. Eventually, the yoga of Niguma is bound to bring practitioners toward this result—not just for their own personal benefit, but for the benefit of all sentient beings.

Acknowledgments

His Holiness the Fourteenth Dalai Lama

Of course, during the 1960s and '70s, there were many changes throughout the world, but this was especially the case for the Tibetan and Chinese people during the Cultural Revolution. So many individuals went through great suffering during this period. Some lost their lives, while others underwent immense hardship and cataclysmic change. Some even lost their country. During this period, however, many tens of thousands of individuals, including great enlightened beings, came to reside in India, Nepal, and Bhutan, and I wholeheartedly acknowledge all those who have carried on their great dedication and determination to the path of Dharma with their inner circle and all of their students.

Above all, I wish to acknowledge His Holiness the Fourteenth Dalai Lama, who for many decades has traveled around the world spreading kindness and compassion and exemplifying the deep meaning of the Buddha's teachings.

We are very fortunate to have a Buddhist teacher of such stature who is so close to us and so relatable. Understand that if there is an enlightened being who is not relatable to all beings, their benefit to resolve the great suffering in the world is much diminished. The Buddha became very famous because he was relatable, not just because he shared the universal truth, including the truth of our illusory body and mind, and how we can better understand them so we may progress along the spiritual path. Therefore, I see His Holiness the Fourteenth Dalai Lama as the present manifestation of the enlightened, historical Buddha Shakyamuni.

The Wangchuk Dynasty and Family

In the 1960s, at the invitation of the Royal Family, the previous Kalu Rinpoche resided in Bhutan and was able to establish a monastic and lay community in the eastern part of the country, and he met many great masters there. Eventually, he went to India, and then traveled around the world establishing many more monasteries, Dharma centers, and retreat centers—and in the process, he cultivated a great many students. Deep gratitude is offered to the Wangchuk Dynasty and family, and especially to the fourth and fifth kings of Bhutan. Throughout history there have been many emperors, kings, and queens. Some have been motivated by their own personal benefit, others for the purpose of gaining reputation and influence. However, I have personally observed the fourth and fifth kings of the Wangchuk Dynasty to have dedicated their entire lives to bodhichitta—the enlightened mind of altruism—and great compassion. They have been thoroughly and wholeheartedly dedicated to keeping the Dharma pure and avoiding divisive politics at every opportunity. They have also maintained the Dharma in the sense of *samaya*, or sacred pledge, and the sense of discipline not just for the country of Bhutan but also for the rest of the world. I have observed that. I have witnessed their wholehearted care for the people who come into Bhutan. But not just that—they also demonstrate compassion in action by offering loving care for the generations to come. The fourth and fifth kings are true examples of Dharma kings. I pray for the longevity of the fourth and fifth Dharma kings of Bhutan and all of the members of the Royal Family from the depth of my heart and with my deepest respect and love.

Tai Situ Rinpoche

I would like to offer acknowledgment to my guru, Tai Situ Rinpoche, who has been loving and caring, not just in building a religious bubble in my head but in giving me freedom to explore and make mistakes. He has always been patient in his guidance. I will be forever grateful to my mentor and guru. He gave me not just Dharma teachings and transmissions, but also showed me the importance of the unique qualities possessed by each individual. The causes and conditions that make up each of us are unique and there is no need to try to appear any differently than we truly are. My guru Tai Situ Rinpoche taught me to be noble, to be honest, to be truthful. All of the tricky games out in the world may make us think we have won, but that is only temporary. Tai Situ Rinpoche taught me to stick to the truth and to focus on compassion. He gave me this guidance for the mundane world, for which I am deeply grateful. Additionally, all of our actions occur in time and over time, and time itself is something we cannot we regain. In this context, I feel so grateful for Tai Situ Rinpoche's generosity; he gave me so much of his time, and because of that, I can see further and more clearly. The faith and trust he has in me is something that I could not even see in myself, but gave me confidence and blessings. My love and devotion is forever with him in this life, as it was in in my previous life.

Buddha Shakyamuni, Niguma, Sukhasiddhi, Khyungpo Naljor

Buddha Shakyamuni, Niguma, Sukhasiddhi, Khyungpo Naljor—each of these historical figures achieved profound realization and compassionately dedicated their lives to transmitting their treasures in a living stream from generation to generation. As the result of the dedication of our forbearers we today have an opportunity to engage in lineage practices and in turn pass on the precious Dharma. Without this spiritual heritage being passed on to the modern day, even if we wanted the living stream to flow through us onto the next generation, we would not have full access to the pure and detailed teachings of our spiritual ancestors, and so the lineage would end with us. Because it comes to us fully intact, we have an immense responsibility to keep it intact and resolve not to be the broken link in a long chain.

My Father and Bokar Rinpoche

My late father and Bokar Rinpoche are two figures who have been very important to me; one of them looked after me until I was seven years old and the other looked after me from that time on, including during my three-year retreat, when I had no else to fill that role. Both of them passed away much too young. Our personal connection was so special, and nothing can replace that. Of course, there was pain throughout my lifetime, but because of their presence in my life, I knew I was held, and that has remained with me until the present moment. The more I travel throughout the world to teach the Dharma and nurture my centers, the more I understand why my late father was so often absent when I was a kid. As the nephew and secretary of the previous Kalu Rinpoche, he too carried immense responsibilities and felt no choice but to shoulder them. Having honed my awareness and concentration in retreat, I am able to appreciate the love, devotion, and connection between the previous Kalu Rinpoche and the previous Bokar Rinpoche as well. As challenging as it has been at times, with obstacles especially early on and enormous responsibility, had I the opportunity to relive my life, I would again choose the path I have taken. This is in large part the result of my deep connection with my father and Bokar Rinpoche and their unshakable bond to my predecessor, the previous Kalu Rinpoche.

Wangchen Rinpoche

Wangchen Rinpoche was deeply dedicated to my predecessor during his youth. He is a close, dear friend who has always been at my side through the inevitable ups and downs, and to this day remains unconditionally supportive.

Michele Loew

Michele Loew is a seasoned hatha yoga instructor, yoga therapist, Vajrayana practitioner, and Vajrayana yoga instructor. She has taught extensively throughout the world and is a student of His Holiness the Fourteenth Dalai Lama, Ling Rinpoche, the Forty-Second Sakya Trizin, myself, and Bob Thurman. She has brought her hatha yoga expertise and comparative study of Niguma yoga with me into this text to help new students prepare to practice the yoga of Niguma. She has contributed to ensuring the correct presentation of important sketches for both hatha yoga and the yoga of Niguma throughout the book, as illustrated by Mia Scarpetta. Michele has also taken great care to ensure that the descriptions of each posture are clear, correct, and readily understandable. I am grateful to her commitment to the practice of yoga, Dharma, and teaching the practice to others.

Wisdom Publications

I would like to acknowledge Daniel Aitken, publisher of Wisdom Publications, and his energetic passion for this book, and Brianna Quick, who has worked tirelessly and skillfully on the front line as a primary editor. She is so skilled in her field and so joyously heartful in her work. I would also like to thank the entire Wisdom team for its support, kindliness, hard work, and skillful means. I am also deeply grateful that they have made the related video segments available online for the benefit of many. It is without question that their chief priority is only the Dharma and its accurate and expert transmission.

Lama Sarah Harding

Lama Sarah Harding has made an invaluable contribution to my journey. Her continued dedication as a practitioner, translator, and supporter of the previous Kalu Rinpoche paved the way for my being here with you now. She and her family sponsored and supported my predecessor in a comprehensive way. Among the karmic fruits of her dedication is that the three-year retreat equally available for men and women was born. I would also like to express my gratitude for all of her translations of Dharma texts with dedication and accuracy. Thank you, and please continue.

Robert Thurman and Michael Kurth

I am grateful to Bob Thurman for putting me in touch with Wisdom Publications. I would like to thank him for all of his work for Tibetan youth and culture and for the Dharma. Michael, thank you for introducing me to Bob. Please accept my deepest gratitude.

You, the Reader

With regard to acknowledgments, while there are many people responsible for making this book possible, I would like to acknowledge you, my dearest reader. Life can seem very long, with misery and joy woven together. It may also seem quite short, with the distractions we experience from all of our senses, including our busy, thinking mind. By memorializing a transmission to you by means of this book, the hope is that my experience with the yoga of Niguma becomes unbound by my own time and place. My true purpose in writing this book is to offer the little experience that I have so that readers can interpret and engage in these practices in precisely the right way, based on their dynamic capacity and existing state of awareness. I wish to acknowledge you, my dear reader, who is making the effort to transform both body and mind through the practice of Niguma yoga.

Some of you may be reading this book out of curiosity. That too is absolutely wonderful because there is no spiritual understanding without curiosity. However, there is a distinction between being completely doubtful and acting with curiosity. Curiosity brings engagement along with questions and ultimately answers during the progression of one's spiritual practice. In this way, the clarity and sharpness of the mind increases over time. On the other hand, if you are always in a state of doubt, you simply remain stuck in the same spot. As such, I am most grateful that you are showing genuine and sincere interest on the journey along the path of Niguma yoga.

Since I have gotten your attention with a special acknowledgment, although we may have never met, I sincerely hope the opportunity arises for us to have an open exchange on meditation and Niguma yoga. I greatly aspire to that.

Appendix:
Supportive Hatha Yoga Postures

HIP OPENING PRACTICES TO SUPPORT YOUR NIGUMA YOGA PRACTICE AND BUILD THE VAJRA POSTURE

Below are the important steps for proper technique in moving into the vajra posture. To prevent injuries and prepare to safely attempt the pose, practice the postures that follow as well as the standing postures presented earlier in the book for knee stability and hip mobility. See also baddha konasana on page 93.

Vajra Posture (Lotus Pose)

Note: You can practice with the left or right leg on top. Traditionally, the left leg folds first in Niguma yoga, but it is fine to have the right leg on top first if that feels better.

Moving into the Pose

1. From a seated position with legs outstretched, lean back and bend your left leg to close the knee joint.
2. While still leaning back, let the left leg fall out to the side. Take hold of the underside of the leg and foot with both hands.
3. Manually move the flesh of the calf toward your pelvis and then up toward the sky. This allows the shin to externally rotate and the top of the shin to turn toward the floor. The shinbone, called the tibia, needs to externally rotate to avoid irritating the knee's medial meniscus. If you grab the leg from

the top to pull it into your pose, you run the risk of straining your knee, as it is the incorrect rotation of the shinbone.

4. Swing your left knee forward and place a relaxed left foot into your right hip crease.

5. Still leaning back with the thighs up off the ground, take the right leg from underneath and do the same swing and external rotation of the tibia to place your foot into the left hip crease.

6. Lower the legs to the ground and come to a neutral position of the pelvis.

7. Sit for a breath or two, particularly when you're first learning, and then move to a simple cross-legged seat or half lotus.

8. Practice hip opening and preparatory poses consistently to maintain flexibility in this pose.

Preparatory Poses and Props

- Janu sirsasana, baddha konasana, ardha baddha padma paschimottanasana, figure four poses, and pigeon pose.
- If there is mild discomfort in the lotus pose, try placing a folded washcloth in the knee crease tightly to assist in compression and the external rotations of the thigh and calf.
- Elevate the pelvis on a folded blanket or cushion to assist the slight anterior tilt of the pelvis and allow the knees to relax down toward the floor. Practice this each day for a few breaths or as long as is comfortable. Do not use this elevation for Niguma yoga practice however, because when you are practicing beps or poses that require standing up and returning to a cross-legged seat on the ground, the landing must always be done on a flat surface. The thighs and pelvis need to touch down to the ground evenly. Landing on anything but flat ground is dangerous.

Precautions and Contraindications

Be cautious for knee tear, particularly the meniscus. Any knee pain is a sign to not do the pose. Ankle strain is also a risk from this pose.

APPENDIX: SUPPORTIVE HATHA YOGA POSTURES   159

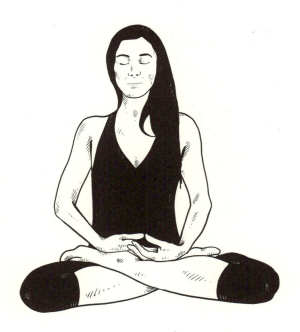

Preliminary Techniques and Preparatory Poses for the Vajra Posture

Variations of the Figure Four Pose

As we have previously discussed, the figure four pose is one of the best practices for beginners and for opening tight outer hip muscles. See page 92 for the supine version of the figure four pose. This seated version of the pose is another excellent method to open the hips and gain the flexibility to engage more fully in the vajra posture.

Seated Figure Four Pose

Moving into the Pose

1. Sit on the floor and lean back like you're getting ready to recline, with the hands behind the pelvis.
2. Cross the right ankle on the left thigh, close to but not on the knee.
3. Dorsiflex the foot to keep the stretch in the hip and glutes and not the knee.

4. Lift your heart and roll your shoulders onto the back. Push with your hands to straighten the spine as much as possible. This will increase the stretch at the hip.

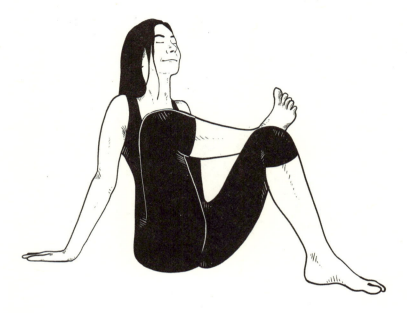

Supta Padangusthasana (Reclined Leg Stretching on the Back)

Students who are feeling stiff in their practice will benefit most from stretching while lying down rather than while seated. Stretching the back of the legs while lying down with a yoga strap or belt in the supta padangusthasana pose is a great way to open up the body to enable ease in Niguma yoga. If you find your lower back sore from sitting practice, that's a good sign you need to stretch these back body muscles and/or the hip flexors more.

Moving into the Pose

1. Lie on your back with your legs together. Legs are active, with the sheaths of the legs drawn in and up, and quadriceps, glutes, and hamstrings contracting vibrantly.
2. Place your left hand on your left thigh.

3. Keeping the left leg active, with the knee cap pointing straight up and the back of the left thigh pressing toward the floor, raise the right leg, catching hold of the big toe with the first two fingers of the right hand. As the leg comes up, it resists the pull of the arm in order to keep an anterior pelvic tilt. Use a yoga strap or belt if you can't catch the foot and keep a neutral spine.

4. Press into the right heel and ball of the foot as you straighten the leg. Raise the leg up until you feel a good stretch that is balanced between effort and ease, and breathe into the belly of the hamstring.

5. Keep the right shoulder grounded, so both shoulders are down and broad. Keep the spine long, with the base of the head broad and open and the chin neutral. Keep the hips relatively squared and the sides of the waist equally long.

6. Stay in the pose for five to ten breaths or longer and then change legs and repeat.

Variations

Chin to Shin: Lift the chin to the shin, engaging the abdominal muscles in a sit-up, and press the lower back into the floor. There is a subtle oblique curl and twist toward the lifted straight leg.

Parsva (Out to the Side): Rotate the right leg externally and move the leg to the side, leading with the toes. Then, once down, slightly bring in the internal rotation pattern by dropping the pubic bone. This will allow the heel to move closer to the ground. When moving into the pose, you can let the pelvis lift on the left side. But once your right leg has come to the floor, turn on the left inner thigh and re-ground your pelvis.

Parivrtta (Twisting Across the Body): Hold onto the right foot with your left hand. Bring the leg across just until the right side of the pelvis begins to lift off the floor and then stop and pull the leg toward your head. Use your right thumb in the hip crease to open your hip. This is an amazing outer hip opener.

Props

- Yoga strap: If you are stiff, use a strap to catch your foot. Place the strap just below the ball mound of your raised leg's foot. The strap will help you stretch and allow you to keep your shoulders down and your spine aligned so you don't have to hunch to catch your toes.
- Foot to wall: It is important to engage the muscles of the leg that is on the ground to keep it neutral and avoid letting it fall out to the side. Until your leg is stronger, you can position your body a leg's distance away from a wall, with the sole of your foot pressing into it to provide muscular support.
- Sandbag on top of straight leg's thigh: If you have a sandbag, use it to weight down the leg on the floor to assist you in keeping it rooted. Pressing the thigh down will ensure your spine stays neutral and you stretch the leg in a balanced way. This prop is particularly nice if you will be stretching for a longer period.

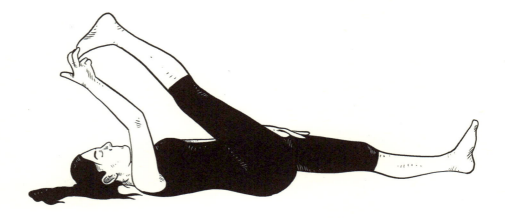

Janu Sirsasana (Head-to-Knee Pose)

The janu sirsasana pose from hatha yoga builds the vajra posture, or lotus pose, and should be practiced until one has ease in folding over completely, with the knee resting firmly on the ground. It is also practiced in Niguma yoga sequence 4. Spending time in this pose daily will allow you to establish the external rotation of the thigh bone needed at the hip joint to move into the vajra posture, as well as bring flexibility to the legs and entire back body. Holding the pose for five to ten breaths or more reduces the stress hormone cortisol, brings in the relaxation response, calms the nervous system, increases parasympathetic response, and improves digestion.

Moving into the Pose

1. Lean back with a posterior tilt to your pelvis and fold your right leg tightly closed, using both hands to create closure at the knee joint. Leaning back allows for the tightest closure of the knee joint, which is essential for the health of the knee.

2. If there is a gap at the knee crease, you can place a folded washcloth in a triangle shape tightly between the calf and knee.

3. Take the folded right leg out to the side and place the sole of the foot to the inseam of your straight left leg.

4. Shift the hips to square to even up the pelvis. To facilitate that, you can lift the straight leg's sit bone up and drag the leg back until your hips are square.

5. Twist your torso to the left and wrap the right waist toward the straight left leg. Twisting toward the straight leg is important to open the hips as well as protect the sacroiliac joint from strain.

6. If the bent knee is off the ground, you can place a firm cushion or block underneath the knee for support.

7. Engage the left quadriceps and press the left leg into the ground. Inhale, lift your arms up high into the air, and lengthen the torso, side body, and spine as much as you can. Exhale and forward fold, catching the foot with the hands or a yoga strap or belt.

8. In the final form, hold the left foot with the palms facing out. The right hand will grab the left wrist, which allows you to leverage spinal extension. Stay for five breaths or more.

9. After you become adept at the pose and feel at ease, begin practicing the half lotus with a forward fold; the pose ardha baddha padma paschimottanasana

is one of the best postures to prep for full lotus once you are able to do janu sirsasana well.

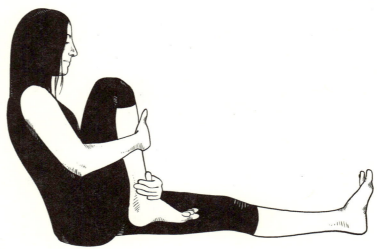

Variation

Parsva janu sirsasana: The fourth image here is a lateral bend variation. Aside from bending to the side, which is done often in Niguma yoga postures, you can also bend forward between the straight leg and knee to stretch your adductors, the inner thigh muscles.

Supta Eka Pada Raja Kapotasana (Reclined Pigeon Pose)

Moving into the Pose

1. From a position with hands and knees on the ground, or down-dog, place the right knee near your right wrist and your right foot near your left wrist. The angle of the shin will depend on what feels good to your knee and body. Angling your shin back, closer to the opposite hip, will require less external rotation and often feels better on the knee because it closes the joint. Because the top of the shin is turned down with the sole of the foot turned up and the foot pointed, it is the classic form that builds one's vajra posture. You can also work with a flexed foot if your shin is parallel to the top of the mat in a figure

APPENDIX: SUPPORTIVE HATHA YOGA POSTURES 165

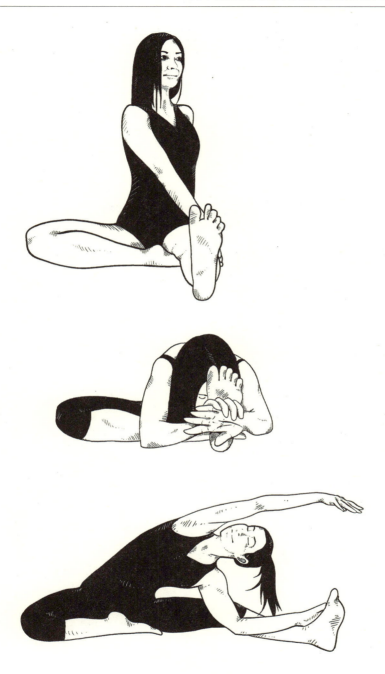

four leg position, but it is generally much harder and will require more elevation if you're stiffer. Try to practice different angles to get into different parts of the hip.

2. Extend the back leg as far back as you can walk it, and lower the pelvis closer to the ground.
3. If your hip flexors are tight, you will need to prop your pelvis higher to alleviate pull on your lower back.
4. If your outer hips are tight, you will need to place padding under the front hip.
5. Inhale and isometrically pull in toward the midline and extend the spine. Keep the length and begin to fold forward until you feel the perfect place to rest and stretch.
6. Send deep breaths from the belly into the hip and pelvis.
7. To finish, exhale and engage the legs before inhaling and lifting up out of the pose.

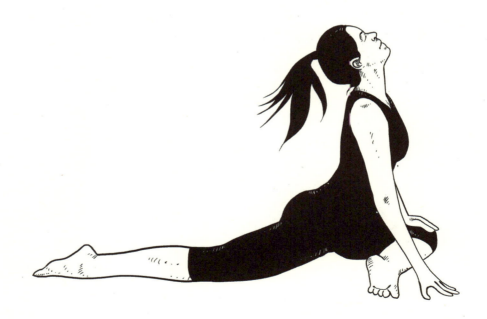

Additional Resources

THE YOGA OF NIGUMA

Video resources to support your practice of the yoga of Niguma are available online, including demonstrations of the twenty-five sequences of Niguma yoga and supporting hatha yoga poses. Please visit www.wisdomexperience.org/niguma-yoga-poses-kalu-rinpoche.

ONLINE COURSES

The Illusory Body and Mind: In this online course, Kalu Rinpoche delves deep into Vajrayana practice as he shares the teachings of numerous pioneers of the Shangpa lineage, including Niguma, Sukhasiddhi, Tangtong Gyalpo, Taranatha, and Jamgon Kongtrul Lodro Thaye. You'll be guided through an introduction to two key completion stage practices from among Niguma's six yogas: the illusory body and mind and bardo (intermediate state) practices.

www.wisdomexperience.org/illusory-body-mind/

Niguma's Dream Yoga: This course builds on the illusory body and mind teachings of Kalu Rinpoche's first course while also moving into teachings and guided practices for dream yoga and more. This course presents another powerful opportunity to receive deeply authentic and inspiring teachings from a remarkable teacher.

https://wisdomexperience.org/nigumas-dream-yoga/

Save 15% on these courses with code KALUBOOK.

About the Authors

His Eminence the Second Kalu Rinpoche is a world-renowned spiritual teacher and emissary of Vajrayana Buddhism. He is lineage holder of the Shangpa tradition, which originated from two female yoginis a thousand years ago. His face-to-face, published, and online teachings have brought to life these previously secretive practices, offering public access to those poised for profound transformation.

He was born on September 17, 1990, in Darjeeling, India. His father, Lama Gyaltsen, was a nephew of the previous Kalu Rinpoche and had also been his secretary since his youth. The Second Kalu Rinpoche was recognized on March 25, 1992, by Tai Situ Rinpoche.

On February 28, 1993, Kalu Rinpoche was inducted into Samdrub Darjay Chöling (Sonada). When his father passed away in 1999, he asked to live in the monastery of Bokar Rinpoche. In 2004, he began a traditional three-year retreat. In 2009, he received from Tai Situ Rinpoche all the transmissions of the Shangpa lineage. On this occasion, he was conferred the cycle of initiations of the lineage 108 times.

In 2010, Kalu Rinpoche traveled to the West for the first time and took charge of the meditation centers the First Kalu Rinpoche had created around the world. In 2014, he returned to Palden Shangpa La Boulaye in France, and in 2019, he returned to the United States to resume the tradition of the Shangpa Monlam initiated by his predecessor.

Having experienced his own challenges along the way, Rinpoche is extraordinarily relatable, kind, and without judgment.

Michele Loew is an international yoga teacher and practitioner of hatha and Vajrayana yogas. Since 1999, she has built community spaces dedicated to the practice of yoga and spirituality. She is the founder of The Yoga Space in Portland, Oregon, as well as the Vajra Yoga School of Comparative Buddhist & Indic Yoga Studies, where she teaches alongside Robert A.F. Thurman, for Tibet House US.

In 2019, she began Clearlight Yoga, her school focusing on yoga nidra and the sleep and dream yoga practices of the Himalayan masters.

She is known as a teacher's teacher, and her yoga schools have been respected by students worldwide for teaching lineage-based yoga focusing on the deeper philosophical and esoteric aspects of the practice, while bringing in cutting-edge modern science and kinesiology into the practice of asana, pranayama, and meditation.

She took refuge with His Holiness the Fourteenth Dalai Lama in 2014 at the Kalachakra Empowerment in Ladakh, India. She continues to study with him as her root guru, and is also a student of the Forty-Second Sakya Trizin, Ling Rinpoche, and of course Kalu Rinpoche.

She serves on the board of directors of Tibet House US and leads retreats and workshops internationally with an altruistic intention to serve and inspire all to discover their enlightened nature. Follow her on social media and online at www.micheleloew.com.

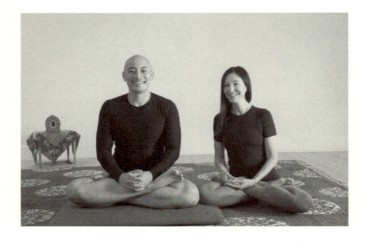

TAKE YOUR PRACTICE DEEPER WITH

The Illusory Body and Mind and Niguma's Dream Yoga

THE WISDOM ACADEMY ONLINE COURSES WITH

H. E. Kalu Rinpoche

✶ **Save 15%** on either (or both!) courses with code **KALUBOOK** ✶

Learn more and begin your journey:
wisdomexperience.org/illusory-body-mind
wisdomexperience.org/nigumas-dream-yoga

✶ About the Courses ✶

H. E. Kalu Rinpoche possesses a remarkable ability to convey the true power and possibility of the Dharma. His Wisdom Academy online courses provide a precious opportunity to receive some of the most profound teachings of Buddhism as they're illuminated and explained by a remarkable teacher. Rinpoche masterfully brings together his deep knowledge of Dharma and his clear, compassionate understanding of modern life and the challenges on the path to liberation. Sign up today to get access to these profound resources.

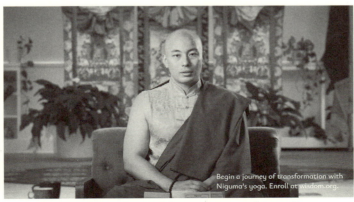

Image: from the Wisdom Academy course Niguma's Dream Yoga

What to Read Next from Wisdom Publications

Luminous Mind

The Way of the Buddha

Kyabje Kalu Rinpoche

"Undoubtedly the best collection of Kalu Rinpoche's teachings. In perusing these pages, I relived the days when I translated for Rinpoche, enthralled by his magical blend of anecdotes, crystal clear explanations, and profound instruction."—Ken McLeod, author of *Wake Up to Your Life*

Tibetan Yoga

Magical Movements of Body, Breath, and Mind

Alejandro Chaoul

Simply put, Alejandro Chaoul's teachings on magical movements are a tremendous gift to yogis everywhere." —Cyndi Lee, founder, OM Yoga

Mindfulness Yoga

The Awakened Union of Breath, Body, and Mind

Frank Jude Boccio

Editor's Choice—*Yoga Journal*

About Wisdom Publications

Wisdom Publications is the leading publisher of classic and contemporary Buddhist books and practical works on mindfulness. To learn more about us or to explore our other books, please visit our website at wisdom.org or contact us at the address below.

Wisdom Publications
132 Perry Street
New York, NY 10014 USA

We are a 501(c)(3) organization, and donations in support of our mission are tax deductible.

Wisdom Publications is affiliated with the Foundation for the Preservation of the Mahayana Tradition (FPMT).